THERE MUST BE MORE TO LIFE THAN THIS . . .

One man's journey on the human side of the statistics and attitudes surrounding obesity in the UK today

STEVE BEER & ALI BAGLEY

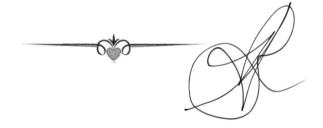

DEDICATION

For those who love us despite our issues, we love you too

For those who struggle silently every day, we feel your pain

For those whose ignorance wounds us, we forgive you

For those who strive for open-mindedness and compassion, we sincerely thank you

Everyone's life journey is theirs to own, and ours to share along the way if we are lucky

CONTENTS

The Must Be More to Life Than This . . . ?

The Must Be More to Life Than This . . . ?

Introduction

Who are we?

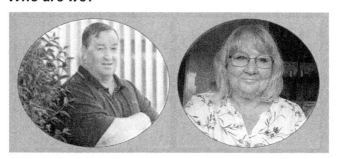

Steve and I are both in lifelong battles against addiction in one form or another. For Steve it began with alcohol and grew into food addiction resulting in chronic health issues, both mental and physical.

For me it has been about food, as a comfort, as a reward, as my friend. Years and years of yoyo dieting, low self-esteem, and ending up morbidly obese from my forties into my fifties.

My point here is that both Steve and I have been there, wherever there is, we got the t-shirt, we walk the talk.

As we write this, we haven't yet got our happy endings, we fight on. The point is we are winning the fight now.

Despite his physical limitations Steve is running his hugely successful podcasts and working with stroke survivors. I am running a very successful business as a Business Impact and Writers coach and have published several business support books including the number one bestseller, Love Coaching, Hate Business.

I am also the Director of an international learning platform based in the methodology of Geo-Emotional Mapping, an innovative way to increase your self-awareness for personal growth and professional development. In this book you will discover this for yourself as we map your relationship with emotional eating.

Why have we written this book?

Steve asked me to help him to tell his story. I work with authors in developing their books from concept to self-publication, so it seemed a fairly usual request.

As it turned out, it was anything but normal. First of all, because of his strokes, Steve is unable to do his own writing, so my first job was to get to know his story and put it together for him in the way he wanted it to be told.

The second job was to find a way to set his story in the context of the statistics and attitudes towards obesity in today's society. So, a lot of research.

The third job was to create a book which not only told Steve's story honestly, authentically and openly, within that context, but also to make it a book that would help others.

Maybe just to let you know that you are not alone, maybe to help you to get onto your own path to recovery, however it could help, we needed it to help.

What are we hoping to change?

In a word: Attitudes

Firstly, we believe that by talking openly about obesity and the deeper emotional issues that contribute to it, by highlighting the stigma associated with it and the often-held assumption that, 'fat people are greedy, lazy and stupid', we can begin to change people's attitudes from hate and ignorance into compassion and understanding.

Secondly, we hope that Steve's story, combined with the interactive sections in each chapter, will help you to change your attitude towards your own issues, to enable you to navigate your journey more successfully from now on.

How this book is structured

Each chapter is dedicated to different life stages, or topics and the statistics (stats), facts, attitudes, issues and stories will be relevant to that stage or topic.

Most chapters have stats and facts, which unless otherwise stated, have come directly from information published by the National Health Service.

We talk about those stats, we ask questions, and we often give our opinions; and opinions is what they are, based on our own knowledge and experiences. You can disagree with us if you want to but please be kind.

And lastly, we have included 'Thought Capture' space for you to write your own learnings and questions. There are also question and answer sections to help you learn more about yourself and your attitudes.

And from the start, we invite you to develop your

own Geo-Emotional map of your relationship with food and obesity through your life's journey.

You can read this book in three different ways:

Way 1: Maybe you are just interested in Steve's story, if so, just read his story, told in his words, on the Steve's Story pages.

Way 2: Maybe you just want to know the stats, facts, info and interactive bits that Ali has written to help you on your own journey. If so, just read the chapters (but we know you want to read Steve's Story too!).

In fact, we know that you are probably going to read both the chapter contents and Steve's story, they go together so why wouldn't you? This is **Way 3:** Enjoy!

We mentioned interactive bits, what are those?

Throughout the book you will find question and answer sections, thoughts capture sections, notes pages and more where you can focus on you and your journey. Ali has used her NLP and Coaching skills to devise these interactive bits to help you become more self-aware about your situation, triggers, needs, and drivers.

Icons

The following icons can be found throughout the book and act as markers to help you jump around the book to get to the interactive stuff you are most interested in. The icons are as follows:

Thought Capture

 Goals & Targets

 Questions & Answers

 Hints, Tips & Ideas

 Geo-Emotional Mapping

 Action Planner

 Where you can find out more

The science bits

In each chapter Ali has included stats and facts from her research into obesity in the UK. Most of the data driving this information comes from the NHS website and publications and was gathered in 2019/2020. These stats and facts are changing all the time so please read them as an indicator and not as being 100% accurate today.

Steve's Story

Almost every chapter begins with Steve's Story, told in his words, and the bits of his story we tell will relate to that chapter specifically.

Sometimes the stories will be hard to read, his journey has not been an easy one and as we write this there is not yet a happy ending.

The Must Be More to Life Than This . . . ?

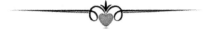

1: Childhood, where our foundations are laid

Steve's Story – Childhood

I am one of four kids, me, Robert, John and Susan. A big family in itself; but add my gran into the mix and that was seven of us, all living together in a three-bedroom flat in the Barbican.

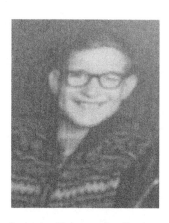

My Dad worked two jobs to support us all, early mornings boiling crabs that my Mum then prepared and sold to the local pubs and restaurants. Then he worked the day for the local council.

So, seven people, small flat, fish, hard work. I was responsibility free, spending my days at Mont Street Primary and evenings at the youth club at Virginia House. Yes, cramped and smelly but full of love and fun. Those happy memories remain with me to this day.

When I was still quite young Mum, Dad, Susan and I moved to our new home in St. Budeaux, near Plymouth. My brothers stayed in the Barbican with Nan. I loved my life in the west country with my family. All in all, my early childhood was great.

In 1981, aged 11, I, like every other eleven-year-old started my time at secondary school. This was something of a culture shock for me. Now I was the youngest kid, a shy kid with a wandering left eye, who smelled of fish, basically I was a target, I might as well have had a sign on my back saying, 'kick me'.

Name calling, bullying, it was tough to deal with and I was miserable. I was a bright kid but a slow learner and when you are in a situation like that it takes over your mind; learning became really difficult for a kid living in fear.

I found myself looking for an escape, a way to deal with what was happening to me, and I found it, by chance, in 1982.

Walking through town, probably up to no good, I found myself walking into St. Andrews church. There was a peacefulness there, it felt like sanctuary for a 12-year-old who needed some calm in his life. I just sat there, in the pew, quietly listening to the sounds of the old building.

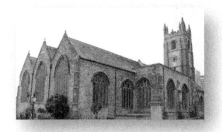

The Minster Church of St Andrew, also known as St Andrew's Church, Plymouth is an Anglican church in Plymouth. It is the original parish church of Sutton, one of the three towns which were later combined to form the city of Plymouth. The church is the largest parish church in the historic county of Devon and was built in the mid to late 15th century. It was designated as a Minster Church in 2009 and it continues to operate as the focus for religious civic events for the city and as a bustling evangelical church.

Coming from one corner of the church I could hear

what sounded like whispering. I was curious so went over to see what it was. There were several people there, on their knees talking quietly with their eyes closed and palms together, praying. I don't know why but I felt compelled to join them. I will never forget how much better I felt afterwards.

A few days later I was in town and again I found myself heading towards the church. It was November and coming up to bonfire night and me and my mate decided that, for fun, we would nick a few bibles to burn on the bonfire (don't judge me, I was 12 and didn't really know any better).

I could hear singing coming from inside. My mate legged it, but I went on in and sat and listened to the music. The choir were a friendly bunch, maybe they could see that this kid needed something even if he couldn't, and they asked me to join them. Before long I was going to the church for choir practice every week, they accepted me, and I felt secure there.

Looking back, joining the choir wasn't about the religion, or celebrating Christ, it was just a means for me to feel that I belonged to something, an interest that kept me off the streets and, in some ways, replicated the days of the Virginia House Youth Club.

It wasn't until 1984, when I was fourteen that Christianity became a force in my life. I went on a church outing to Aston Gate, where the evangelist preacher Billy Graham was speaking. I was entranced by this man and what he had to say. Salvation and love, everything I needed, spoken in a way that connected to my soul. That is how I became a Christian.

My newfound faith didn't exactly help me when it came to school, in fact the smelly kid with the wonky eye now carried a bible around with him. The target on my back was bigger now! Strangely though, my faith acted like a shield against the harsh words and attacks, like a comfort blanket protecting me from the hurt and fear.

My faith in God extended to a new faith in myself and I discovered running and football. I got stronger, physically and mentally. I had this gift from God which saw me running in school cross country mini marathons, full marathons and playing for the football team.

In the bible it says, "Do not worry about your physical well-being. People who don't know any better run after all the things they want, but your Heavenly Father knows your needs. Run for his kingdom and his righteousness then everything that you need will be taken care of."

You see running was my hobby, I was good at it, I won trophies and medals, but I used the running as a comfort, even if it was only for a few minutes it set me apart from the loneliness and the need to be wanted. When I ran, I was free, of fear, of pain, of loneliness.

At the same time, I felt a pull towards school ministry, helping others to find God and the joy of faith. I doubted myself, maybe I was afraid of what people would think, that I was weird or some kind of loon. I had gone through years of bullying at this point, I was mentally scarred from it and my confidence and self-esteem were pretty low. I prayed to God, 'why me, I can't do this'.

Somehow, I found the courage to try and began by

organizing a weekly dinner time get together for the kids to come and learn about faith. I had no idea whether anyone would turn up and for some weeks I sat there alone, waiting, disappointed.

Then one week three people came, Graham, Peter and Stephan. And then the group began to grow and before long we were doing school assemblies and even putting on plays at local youth clubs.

I visited more schools, spreading the word. I wasn't comfortable with it, but I did it and I carry a sense of pride with me that through my efforts many young people were able to find the peace and love that I had found through my faith.

So that was my childhood, happy early years of family love and fun, followed by a new home, bullying, going off the rails, finding Christ, getting back on the rails and making a difference in the life of others. My final challenge as I headed into adulthood and the big wide world was to pass my final exams.

I was a slow learner, not stupid, just slow. I never gave up trying though and, with the help of my Pastor, David Chard, I was able to learn enough about religious education to pass the exam.

I last saw David just before he died in 2002 and I was able to say thank you so much for everything he had done for me in my life. He was not only a minster, he was also a wonderful friend.

1986 - Childhood over, adulthood begun.

Obesity in Childhood

When my daughter was in her early teens, she was very overweight. Looking back (ah the joy of hindsight) maybe I should have paid more attention, been more in control of what she was eating, stopped her from becoming overweight in the first place. Maybe, but I let her down.

Weirdly it was at that time that I was working for Weight Watchers™ and had very much got my weight under control. Was I self-absorbed? Possibly? Is that an excuse? Not really.

I am an intelligent woman, I consider myself to be a good mother, yet I let my little girl overeat to the point where she was clinically overweight.

She tells me that she was bullied very badly during that period (I didn't know that then). Was that because she was overweight, or did she overeat to compensate for the bullying?

My point here is that obesity in children, in my opinion, is very much in the control of the parents, but that even the most switched on and loving parents can struggle to handle it well. And that even the brightest kids can be held hostage to their own negative emotions and difficult life experiences.

Furthermore, there is a link between obesity in children and the BMI of their parents.

It's complex folks. Let's look at the stats and facts

Stats & Facts

From data gathered between April 2019 and December 2020 it was discovered that most children aged between 2 and 15 were neither overweight nor obese: 69% of boys and 73% of girls were normal weight. However, 20% of boys and 13% of girls were obese.

Based on these figures in 2019 it was estimated that 1.6 million children aged between 2 and 15 were obese, including 970,000 boys and 590,000 girls.

It was also found that obesity in children was closely related to their parent's BMI status.

Children were also more likely to be either overweight or obese if their mothers were. 17% of children whose mothers were neither overweight nor obese were overweight or obese, compared with 29% of children whose mothers were overweight but not obese and 44% of those with obese mothers were either overweight or obese themselves.

The association with fathers' BMI was also marked: obesity increased from 8% of children with fathers who were neither overweight nor obese to 23% of those with obese fathers. Similarly, the proportion of children who were overweight or obese increased from 19% of children with fathers who were neither overweight nor obese to 41% of those with obese fathers.

Obesity in children can not only lead to health issues in later life but also whilst still in childhood. In 2019, 613 children under 16 were admitted to hospital in the UK with a primary diagnosis of obesity, in essence the reason for their admission was because of their weight. This was higher than the number for 16-to-24-year-olds in the same time period.

A further 7,186 children under 16 years old had

obesity listed as a secondary diagnosis on admission to hospital that year.

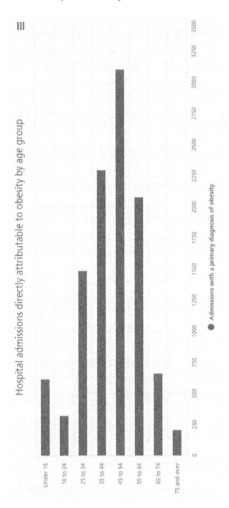

The statistics referred to in this section have been sourced from: https://files.digital.nhs.uk/9D/4195D5/HSE19-Overweight-obesity-rep.pdf and *Hospital Episode*

Statistics (HES), NHS Digital.

The following chart demonstrates the prevalence of overweight and obesity in children, by age: 1995-2019 (three year rolling average):

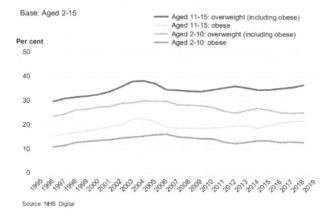

These are the breakdowns specific to 2019

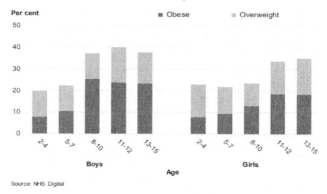

We can see from the following chart that overweight and obesity in children also varies depending on household income, with children from the poorest households being most affected.

The Must Be More to Life Than This . . . ?

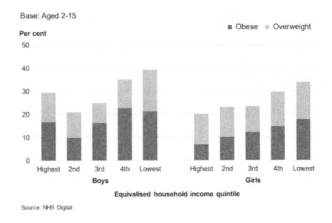

Base: Aged 2-15

Per cent

■ Obese ■ Overweight

Boys / Girls

Equivalised household income quintile

Source: NHS Digital

Add to this the fact that children with overweight and obese parents are more likely to be overweight or obese, and that adults in poorer households are more likely themselves to be overweight or obese and we see an undeniable pattern emerging.

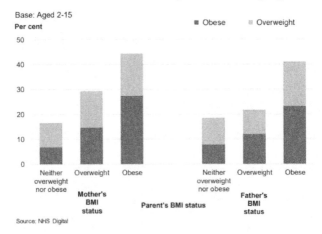

Base: Aged 2-15

Per cent

■ Obese ■ Overweight

Mother's BMI status / Father's BMI status

Parent's BMI status

Source: NHS Digital

If a child lives in a household with overweight / obese parents who are also on a low income, their chances of becoming overweight or obese are much higher than for children living in higher income households with 'normal' weight parents.

Current Thinking & Making Changes

According to the governments guidance document **Childhood obesity: a plan for action** "Today nearly a third of children aged 2 to 15 are overweight or obese and younger generations are becoming obese at earlier ages and staying obese for longer. Reducing obesity levels will save lives as obesity doubles the risk of dying prematurely.

Obese adults are seven times more likely to become a type 2 diabetic than adults of a healthy weight which may cause blindness or limb amputation. And not only are obese people more likely to get physical health conditions like heart disease, but they are also more likely to be living with conditions like depression."

Worryingly this document does not seem to have been updated since 2017, despite a worldwide pandemic and ongoing research into childhood obesity.

We have also seen that the statistics in 2019 there was still an upward trend in obesity amongst 11- to 15-year-olds, a full 2 years after the last update to the plan.

At that time one of the proposed actions was to launch a 'broad, structured sugar reduction program' designed to cut children's sugar intake by 20% by 2020. This program, led and run by Public Health England (PHE) issued a progress report in October 2020.

In that report they publish a table (ES1a) showing the reduction in sugar content, by percentage, of the targeted food groups.

Table ES1a. Summary of change in sugar content by food category

| Product Category | Sugar per 100g | |
	Retailers and manufacturers (% change in SWA[+])	Eating out of home sector (% change in SA[$])
Overall	-3.0	-0.3
Biscuits	-1.6	-3.9
Breakfast cereals	-13.3	-17.1
Chocolate confectionery	-0.4	10.7
Ice cream, lollies and sorbets	-6.4	-2.3
Puddings	2.0	2.4
Sweet spreads and sauces	-5.6	N/A
Sweet confectionery	-0.1	N/A [**]
Yogurts and fromage frais	-12.9	2.4
Cakes	-4.8 [*]	-6.8
Morning goods	-5.6 [*]	-0.4

Notes

+   Sales weighted average is the mean weighted by total sales, giving more influence to products with higher sales

$ Simple average is the simple arithmetic mean. Products are given equal influence. The baseline is 2017

*   The baseline for cakes and morning goods for retailers and manufacturers is 2017 rather than 2015

** Data for sweet confectionery in the eating out of home sector has been excluded due to incomparability of results

The basic summary of findings is that there has been very little change. This is not encouraging.

In the 2017 **Childhood obesity: a plan for action** you can also see a drive to encourage all public sector food and catering services to ensure that the easy choices are healthy choices when it comes to food. That is in hospitals, schools and other similar institutions.

Since 2017 we have also seen the birth of **'The Daily Mile'** initiative. This scheme (https://thedailymile.co.uk/) encourages all children to run or walk a mile every day in order to develop their physical health and mental wellbeing. The scheme now runs in 85 countries with over 3 million children a day joining in.

Whilst I was researching initiatives to reduce childhood overweight and obesity, I found a great site www.eufic.org which includes a table of successful measures to prevent childhood obesity which I reproduce in its entirety below:

Successful Measure	Examples
Facilitate physical activity	Introduce active breaks in schools
Provide easy access to the healthy foods **Eliminate unhealthy foods**	Make contract only with companies providing healthy options for food and drinks options sold and/or provided in schools. Monitor the numbers, content and placement of vending machines. Ensure that safe drinking water is always accessible.
Restrict marketing for unhealthy food	Prohibit all advertising directed at children under 18 years in child welfare and child protection institutions, kindergartens, elementary schools and their dormitories.
Improve education on	Provide nutrition training

nutrition and healthy lifestyle	to teachers and to school kitchen staff.
Care for children with overweight	Measure children's weight and height periodically. Give feedback to children with overweight and their parents with leaflets and online resources to promote healthy lifestyle practices. Insert children affected by obesity a supervised lifestyle program.
Monitor and screen for children have developed overweight	National school-based surveillance system assessing the physical and motor development of children.
Take initiative	In the absence of national or municipal regulation, establish own school policies. Open the schools to parents to make them aware of the pedagogy and be active in the process.

These are great initiatives and if followed through will hopefully begin to reduce the childhood obesity issues we have in the UK.

However, based on the statistics we have seen in this chapter, are we doing enough to educate the parents and guardians of these children? What is the point of initiatives in school if the child then goes home to take-aways, sweets and an evening in front of their games console?

This book does not even attempt to answer that question. Our mission is to highlight that there is a problem and that right now, in our opinion, not enough is being done to tackle it in terms of parental education.

My experience, as a chubby child, was that I didn't know any better and that my parents were overweight, didn't know any better themselves and exercised very little control over what I ate and what exercise I took. That was fifty years ago. Have things changed?

What are your thoughts on the subject of childhood obesity?

Thoughts Capture:

The Must Be More to Life Than This . . . ?

_____

_____

_____

_____

_____

_____

_____

_____

_____

_____

_____

_____

_____

_____

_____

_____

Mapping Your Emotional Relationship with Food

The objective:

Whether you are currently overweight, obese or of a normal weight for your height you will have an emotional relationship with food.

In this section I am going to introduce you to a methodology known as Geo-Emotional Mapping (GEM). The objective of GEM is to give the mapper a third-party perspective on his or her relationship with food. By mapping out your relationship in this way you will be able to disassociate yourself from the emotions and so take an observers view.

This in turn will enable you to see your strengths more clearly, help you to understand where things have not gone so well and in turn help you to make a plan of action to move forward in your journey.

GEM as a methodology can be used for any situation however for this book, we are focusing on using it to map out your relationship with food.

If you would like to know more about GEM, how it works, the different applications for it, even get involved as a 'Geographer of Emotions' like me, then please email me at:
ali@bertagniconsulting.com.

The Instructions

You are going to need a couple of things for this exercise:

1. Plain paper upon which to draw your map/s
2. Pencils, pens, crayons, whatever drawing implements you want to use to create your map.

Now, this map is not an ordinary map, it is not a list of places or events in the usual sense. You are going to be mapping the pivotal events in your relationship with food in terms of your emotions and their corresponding external feature. To do this, you will need 'The Wheels'. (These are trademarked so please do not duplicate these in any way without express permission from Emotional Geography UK Ltd).

The Wheels of Emotions:

The Geographical Elements Wheel:

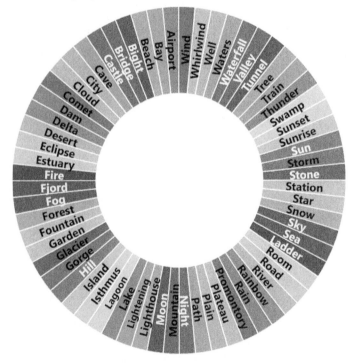

The Emotions Wheel:

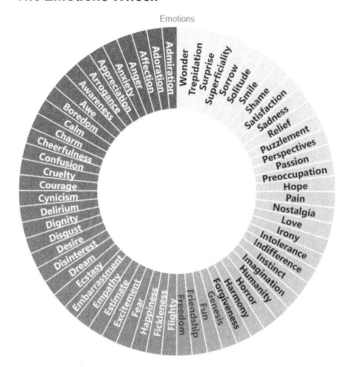

So, what do you do with the wheels?

Here are the instructions:

1. In your mind go back to the first memory you have about food. Focus on that memory by remembering how you felt in that moment.
2. Now give that emotion a name (use the emotions wheel to help you if you need suggestions).
3. Once you have that emotion think about a geographical feature / astronomical / weather element that resonates with how

you felt (use the Geographical Elements
wheel to help you if needed).
4. Now name that pivotal event for your
    emotion and element.

For example: My first memory of food was the
birthday cake at my 5th birthday party. It filled me
with excitement as my Mum brought it out with the
candles flickering on the top and everybody singing
to me. It also made me feel very special but the
emotion I choose to remember that event by is
'Excitement'.

Deciding on a geographical feature that resonates
with that emotion in that event was a little more
difficult, but I settled on 'Garden' because I was in
the garden for my party.

So, my first pivotal event in my relationship with
food was the Garden of Excitement.

5. Now draw a river on your map. It can start
    from the sea, or the source and it can end at
    the sea or the source, or be a circle with no
    beginning or end, it's up to you.
6. Plot your first pivotal event on the map, at
    the beginning of your river, by writing the
    name and drawing your vision of it.

Here is my first section of
my map:

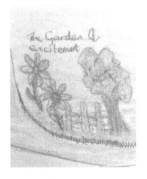

7. Now repeat this for every pivotal event you can bring to mind in relation to your experiences with food during your life.
8. When you are finished, put the map away for at least a day.
9. When you are ready, get the map out and look at it as if you have never seen it before.
10. Now write down your thoughts and observations about the map, capturing any lessons you have learned from the exercise.

My Map Analysis:

_____

_____

_____

_____

_____

_____

_____

_____

_____

_____

_____

The Must Be More to Life Than This . . . ?

The Must Be More to Life Than This . . . ?

_____

_____

_____

_____

_____

_____

_____

_____

_____

_____

_____

_____

_____

_____

_____

_____

_____

What changes are you going to make in your life based on what you have learned?

Action Planner:

You may have discovered many things from your map. You may have had some thoughts about changing your attitude or behaviour towards food or towards people who are obese.

As a result, will you make any changes in your life?

List three key changes you can make to be healthier, slimmer, more tolerant or better informed as you more forwards:

1.

_____

_____

_____

2.

_____

_____

_____

3.

_____

_____

_____

Ali's River of Food Map

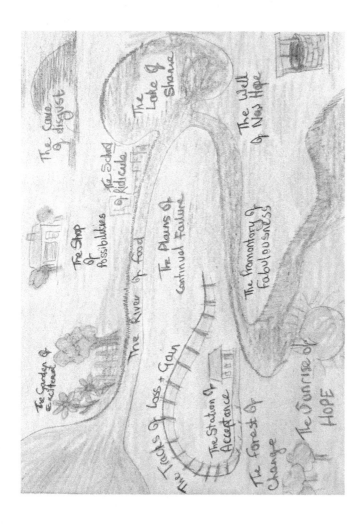

The Must Be More to Life Than This . . . ?

2: Young Adult – addictions, changes and trying to fit in

Steve's Story - Falling Down

The end of 1986 saw the beginning of a downward spiral that was to last for many, many years.

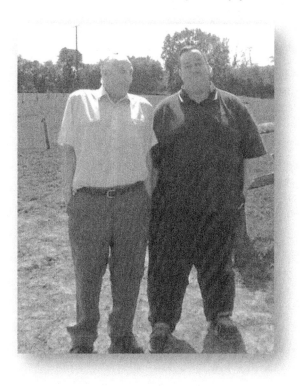

My Dad was a drinker, but he wasn't a nice drunk and my mum and us kids suffered a lot of aggression from him because of it. I was 16 when I started drinking with him and it wasn't long before I started showing the same patterns of behaviour.

I started going into pubs and clubs with my dad who was a 7 days a week drinker. It was a horrible time when I often saw mum beaten up and abused by him.

I didn't want to get drunk, I liked the social side of meeting friends and having fun but I was soon drinking way to much, sleeping on the sofa and living a life I wanted to escape from.

When I was 17 I moved into a friends flat nearby and for a while everything was ok.

Looking back, I can't say whether I started drinking with him because of pressure from him or because I wanted to be more 'grown up'. Whatever the reason I slipped into that addiction very quickly and my life began to go downhill from there on in.

It's worth stating that I was not obese back then, I was a fit healthy young man, not too bad looking, and the drinking didn't have much of an impact on my weight because I was really active.

By the time I was 18 I was married. I had a real problem with alcohol, and this manifested in my violence towards my wife. After 6 months the marriage was over. I think that I lost my faith during that time, both in God and myself. I was a horrible, violent alcoholic who was totally self-absorbed.

It was some time after we broke up that I discovered that she had been pregnant at the time. I tried to make amends and get us back together, but it was too late, it was over.

It was however the shakeup I needed to realise that I needed to get help. Thankfully I was able to go into rehab in Paignton, three months of hard work, but I came out much better.

Still in my early twenties, divorced, a child I hadn't met and now in rehab. It wasn't a great start and the long-term negative impact on my confidence and wellbeing was starting to take hold.

After rehab I got a job, a new girlfriend and before long we were married with two kids, and everything seemed to be going great until she told me that she was leaving me, with the kids, for her cousin, my childhood friend since we were 2 years old.

Downward spiral again. This time I had lost my wife, my kids, my home. I was medicated for depression but soon found myself admitted to Moorfields Acute Unit, a psychiatric hospital. Being in a ward with five people, my Mum telling me she couldn't understand what was going on with me and having lost everything, felt like the end of the world for me.

Through all this my faith in God remained and I was able, with his help to recover and get back out into the world again. Two more marriages, two more failures. No contact with my children, I was no good at relationships.

The more I 'failed' the more I sought comfort in food. Thus began, in my twenties and early thirties, a toxic relationship between me and eating and declining health which would ultimately bring me right to the edge of sanity.

Addiction in Young Adults

Why do young people become addicted, either to drugs, alcohol or food? You might as well ask, how long is a piece of string.

There are many studies and research into this question that constantly bring us back to the issue of mental health when it comes to addiction.

Like the chicken and the egg scenario, does addiction start with poor mental health or does addiction cause poor mental health. Well probably both.

There are certainly many ways that drugs, alcohol and overeating can impact on mental health.

Some people may use these as a way of dealing with difficult feelings and emotions. Young people especially are dealing with heightened emotions that they cannot always understand or control. It is a time of extraordinary emotional and physical change, no wonder kids look for some kind of crutch to help them through it.

Difficult to handle and understand feelings may come from stressful, upsetting or abusive experiences they have gone through. They may be linked directly to a mental health problem; whatever the reason young people turn to addiction, it usually makes those emotions feel even more intense and this can have a negative impact on their mental health.

When people reach a point where they feel like the drug/alcohol/food is in control, maybe using it in secret, away from friends, and life revolves around getting more of it, then you have a real problem. This is how becoming addicted begins.

Add the risk that abusing drugs, drinking too much or overeating could make a mental health condition worse – or make someone more likely to develop one. For instance, there's a strong link between cannabis use and paranoia and psychosis. Other drugs such as LSD and magic mushrooms can make you physically very ill, cause you to hallucinate or have flashbacks, or even kill you.

Having a mental health problem that affects a person's judgement might make them even more likely to turn to addictive behaviour and engage in taking other types of risks.

If you are a young adult, thinking about taking drugs, maybe realising that you are drinking too much or are eating more than is healthy for you on a regular basis then it's really important to know what effect this can have on your body. Speak to your GP about it and how it could affect any mental health medications you may be taking.

 Go through the Question and Answer section later in this chapter to see if you may be experiencing addiction.

 https://www.youngminds.org.uk/young-person/coping-with-life/drugs-and-alcohol/

Stats & Facts

According to https://digital.nhs.uk/data-and-information/publications/statistical/statistics-on-drug-misuse/2019/part-4-drug-use-among-young-people, on the first occasion school age children took drugs, they were most likely to say they did so 'to see what it was like' (50%), whilst on the most recent occasion they were most likely to say 'to get high or feel good' (42%).

According to https://www.gov.uk/government/statistics/substance-misuse-treatment-for-young-people-statistics-2019-to-2020/young-peoples-substance-misuse-treatment-statistics-2019-to-2020-report, there were 14,291 young people (aged under 18) in contact with alcohol and drug services between April 2019 and March 2020. This is a 3% reduction on the number the previous year (14,777) and a 42% reduction on the number in treatment since 2008 to 2009 (24,494). This number is still way too high.

When we look at the figures around alcohol and substance addiction in young adults the figures begin to rise steeply from age 20 up to a peak between the ages of 35 to 39.

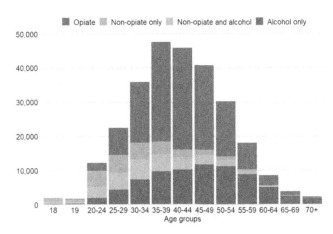

Sourced from: https://www.gov.uk/government/statistics/substance-misuse-treatment-for-adults-statistics-2019-to-2020/adult-substance-misuse-treatment-statistics-2019-to-2020-report

These figures refer only to people in treatment for their addictions, calculating how many people are addicted in total is an impossible task.

One statistic I noted from the figures reported was that in every type of addiction there was a more than 50% need for mental health support but that 25% of those people were not receiving the necessary support.

When it came to researching food addiction, there was much less information to be found.

 According to https://www.priorygroup.com/eating-disorders/eating-disorder-statistics, "Eating disorders, including anorexia nervosa, bulimia nervosa, binge-eating disorder (BED) and other specified feeding or eating disorder (OSFED), which may also be known as 'eating disorders not otherwise specified (EDNOS)', are responsible for more loss of life than any other mental health condition, and unfortunately, are becoming increasingly more common. Over the last 30-40 years, the prevalence of eating disorders has increased to become a widespread problem across the UK and worldwide."

Now this refers to eating disorders, not specifically food addiction. Information on that was really hard to find. Is this because the statistics relate mainly to obesity (one result of food addiction) or because it is not recognized as an 'addiction' as such?

The Priory Group talk about people with BED (Binge Eating Disorder) as those who may use binge eating as a way to cope with mental health problems such as depression, anxiety, or stress.

This binging often causes sufferers to experience intense feelings of guilt, disgust, and low self-esteem and in addition, compulsive overeating tends to happen in secret.

For example, individuals with BED may eat a normal amount of healthy food throughout the day and in public, but then binge eat at night in secret. Therefore, even if these people become overweight, others may not be able to understand why.

The official NHS stats around obesity can be found in Chapter 1, stats around food addiction are impossible to calculate, possibly in part due to the secretive nature of the addiction.

Ultimately, eating causes pleasure hormones to be released in the brain, and we become hooked on those pleasurable feelings. As with other types of addiction, food obsession can destroy a person's life unless they are unable to break away from the behaviour.

Current Thinking & Making Changes

So, what is being done to help people to overcome their addictions to food and the resulting suffering when those people become obese?

As mentioned in more detail in Chapter 3, my addiction to food began as a comfort mechanism to deal with abuse in my first marriage. Steve's began as a way of dealing with his relationship breakdowns and his perceived failure to maintain good relationships.

Steve tells of the times he has been spat at in the street and called horrible names, just because he is fat. In the end he became afraid to leave his home.

The point I am making here is that in order to make changes we need to be aware of the causes and scale of the problem and with obesity that is very difficult for many reasons, such as:

- The secretive nature of the addiction

- The easy availability of unhealthy foods, home delivery takeaways, prepacked microwave meals and so on

- The multitude of causes of the problem that vary so much between individuals and in different cultures

- The difficulty in losing weight once gained

- The lack of healthy eating education, particularly in deprived communities

- It often begins in childhood

It is so much easier to come home after a long day at work, order a pizza and relax in front of the TV than it is to come home, cook a meal using fresh ingredients and take some exercise.

IT IS EASY TO BECOME OVERWEIGHT

IT IS HARD TO STICK TO A HEALTHY EATING REGIME

IT IS INCREDIBLY DIFFICULT TO LOSE WEIGHT ONCE GAINED

High calorie, high sugar, easy to prepare foods are cheap and readily available. How do we deal with this in order to help people, especially those on low incomes, to live healthier lifestyles?

The government, in my lifetime, have successfully introduced laws to make seatbelts mandatory and smoking in many public places illegal. Should we be campaigning to see similar laws around restricting certain foods and drinks in the UK?

It's not possible to do that because of the enormity of the circumstances around food production and consumption but the following measures have been introduced in recent years:

Public Health England (PHE)

https://www.gov.uk/government/organisations/public-health-england launched a sugar reduction and wider reformulation program through which they planned to engage with all sectors of the food industry to reduce the amount of sugar in the foods that contribute most to children's intakes by 20% by 2020, with a 5% reduction in the first year.

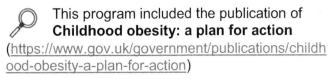 This program included the publication of **Childhood obesity: a plan for action** (https://www.gov.uk/government/publications/childhood-obesity-a-plan-for-action)

As of the 11th of May 2021, the following progress had been made in sugar reduction in the UK between 2015 and 2019:

Retailers and manufacturer branded products

The main findings were:

- overall, there was a 3.0% reduction in the sales weighted average total sugar per 100g in products sold between baseline (2015) and year 3 (2019)

- there were larger reductions for specific product categories, yogurts and fromage frais down 12.9%, and breakfast cereals down 13.3% compared with baseline

- there was a small increase in the puddings category

Eating out of home sector

The main findings were:

- overall, there has been hardly any change in the simple average sugar content from 24.6g per 100g at baseline (2017) to 24.5g per 100g in year 3 (2019) 4

- the largest decreases were 17.1% for breakfast cereals, 6.8% for cakes and 3.9% for biscuits

- there was an increase for chocolate confectionery of 10.7%

For most categories, the simple average sugar content per 100g in products from the eating out of home sector is roughly the same as in retailers and manufacturer branded products in year 3 (2019).

In essence, nothing much has changed in relation to sugar content in foods and furthermore, there has been very little change in the number of calories consumed on a single occasion in the same time period:

Retailers and manufacturer branded products

- overall there has been hardly any change, since 2015, in calories in products likely to be consumed on a single occasion (sales weighted average 146 kcals per portion in 2015 and 147 kcals in 2019)

- there have been some changes at category level; the largest decreases were 7.8% for yogurts and fromage frais, and 3.1% for chocolate confectionery

- the largest increase was 9.0% for puddings

- cakes had an increase of 2.2% and morning goods had an increase of 2.5%, both against a 2017 baseline

In actual fact there has been a 2.6% increase in the tonnes of sugar sold from the product categories included in the program between baseline and year 3. Epic fail.

There is a very clear indication that the problem is understood and there is a willingness to tackle it but moves so far have not been effective.

 More recently PHE have published (July 2020) 'Tackling obesity: empowering adults and children to live healthier lives' https://www.gov.uk/government/publications/tacklin g-obesity-government-strategy/tackling-obesity-empowering-adults-and-children-to-live-healthier-lives

 Information in this section has been sourced from: Sugar reduction and wider reformulation - GOV.UK (www.gov.uk)

What Are Your Addictions?

Think about anything that you feel you cannot do without, why you can't do without it and the impact it has on your wellbeing, physical and mental.

Questions & Answers:

What do you think about before anything else when you wake up in the morning?

_____

_____

_____

Do you have cravings which distract you from normal day to day activities?

_____

_____

_____

Do you spend on more money on food (drugs and / or alcohol than you can afford each week?

_____

_____

_____

When you feel low or stressed what do you do to make yourself feel better?

_____

_____

_____

When you need to focus on study or work, or be more alert, what do you do?

_____

_____

_____

Have people around you suggested that you might have a problem with addiction? If so, how did you feel about that?

_____

_____

_____

Are your friends / colleagues / family members putting pressure on you to behave in a way that you feel is not right for you in relation to food, drugs or alcohol?

_____

_____

_____

Do any of your answers to the above questions give you cause for concern? If so, please seek professional support to address any issues you may have.

What Have You Learned About Yourself?

Thoughts Capture:

_____

_____

_____

_____

_____

_____

_____

_____

_____

_____

_____

_____

_____

_____

_____

_____

_____

_____

_____

_____

_____

_____

_____

_____

_____

_____

_____
_____
_____
_____
_____
_____
_____
_____

What changes are you going to make in your life based on what you have learned?

Action Planner:

Changes I need to make in my life:

1. _____
   _____
   _____

2. _____
   _____

3. _____
   _____

4. _____
   _____
   _____

The Must Be More to Life Than This . . . ?

3: Relationships – the impact when it all goes wrong

Steve's Story – Relationships

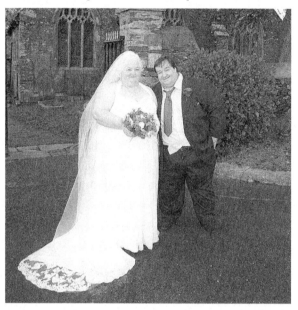

I have had several pivotal relationships in my life, including the relationship with my parents, the support of my pastor David Chard and my six marriages.

I have loved and been loved yet it has been when these relationships have failed, or been lost, that my weight problems have escalated.

I was a fit and healthy man until I lost my mother.

In 2002 I moved home, back in with my parents, after the breakdown of yet another marriage. Six months after returning to Plymouth my mum died. I was there when she was taken by the ambulance. I loved my mum and it was a shock to everyone, but my relationship with my dad was stronger.

I love my dad so much and I did tell him that I loved him. How many of us tell our parents or loved ones how much we love them?

There's always a story behind a weight problem, you don't know what people like me are going through. I don't want to be obese, being so overweight makes it difficult to sleep and I'm too scared to shut my eyes because I worry I won't wake up because of my size. I have to shake my head from side to side to get me off to sleep, to try and get rid of the problems inside my head.

Then I wake up and I'm shattered. I just put my legs up on the sofa and watch TV all day. I have to take anti-depressants and I frequently break down in tears.

I'm happily married to my 6th wife Michelle now, for 7 years, but I am unable to conquer my cravings for junk food. Eating high fat, high sugar foods has become an unbreakable habit for me.

Michelle, and I have been together for 11 years, married 7 years and we have been through a lot. Michelle had children from a previous relationship but because of issues the children were taken away. She went into a downward spiral and was very depressed, it was horrible times. Michelle was pregnant with our child but fell downstairs and we lost the baby. Today we are married, happy and we love each other. We have not got any money saved but we have each other and God. Michelle will be 50 this year but she still beautiful and a lovely wife and yes I am a lucky man.

Michelle loves me and wants me to be happy so

she brings me the foods I crave because I cannot leave the flat we share. She says that, "I find it hard to say no when he asks for food because he nags and nags until I get it. I only go down to the shop for him for a quiet life."

My mental health issues have resulted in years of addiction. Firstly, to alcohol in my early 20s, and then food, resulting in me ending up morbidly obese. I have the classic symptoms of depression including self-harm, suicidal tendencies, attachment & relationship issues. Before Michelle, I found it very difficult to maintain meaningful relationships and I think this is the main reason why I became obese.

Even during my marriage to Michelle, after a disastrous appearance on Channel 5s "Too Fat to Work", the attacks I suffered from the media and the public sent me on a journey of self-destruction that nearly ended up in me attempting to kill myself by jumping off a bridge.

Thankfully I failed and I was sectioned for 72 hours. But when I got home, I carried on self-harming and sank deeper into depression. I was so afraid of attacks that I was unable to leave the flat, to scared to answer the phone, and unable to cope with mounting debt and estrangement from my family.

It wasn't until a year later that I accepted that I had an eating disorder and by seeking help I was finally diagnosed with a borderline personality disorder.

In 2015, we were both determined to lose weight and get healthy when Michelle discovered she was pregnant. Unfortunately, not only did we lose our child through miscarriage, but we lost our motivation and once again I fell back into the cycle of self-abuse and weight gain.

A Poem by Stephen Beer

If you have those doubts
Then let me take it away
If you have those fears
Let me hold you tight
I'm not running away…
I'm not running away…

My heart does always tell
We are meant for each other
Don't want to go somewhere
Without you at my side
I'm not running away…
I'm not running away…

If you have those doubts
Please throw it away
Don't let your fears
Grip you to death
I'm not running away…
I'm not running away…

My heart dictates
We belong together
Promise I won't leave
Without you at my side
I'm not running away…
I'm not running away…

Different Types of Relationships

As you have seen from Steve's story so far, issues in his relationships with his father and his previous wives have often been the basis for his addictions and mental health problems.

We have also seen a statistical relationship between obesity in children and obesity in their parents in the Chapter 1 stats and facts, suggesting that family behaviours can impact through generations.

As human beings we have many different kinds of relationships with people:

- Parents
- Siblings
- Children
- Friends
- Teachers
- Doctors
- Pupils
- Colleagues
- Partners
- Bosses
- Wider Family
- Friends of Friends

To name just a few.

The impact on our mental health, as a result of negativity in these relationships, can be devastating to our general wellbeing and, as in Steve's case, to our weight and physical health.

So, what do we mean by negativity in relationships?

I personally went through a marriage where my then husband tried to cut me off from others so that I was totally dependent on him, and he controlled me. My reaction to that was to make myself feel better with food, which in turn gave him more ways to break my confidence as I got heavier. A vicious circle of control, defiance, mental abuse and control again.

Even today, over thirty years later, I have to work hard at my self-confidence because of the abuse I suffered back then.

Negativity in relationships can also come from yourself. Steve's marriages never lasted, and he believes that he is, 'no good as a husband'. He has 'failed'. To escape those negative feelings, he turned to alcohol initially and later to food.

All of our relationships are different, some very wonderful, others very damaging. Are your relationships damaging your mental wellbeing and impacting on your weight problem?

 Think about this in the Q&A section in this chapter.

Stats & Facts

Both my addictions and Steve's developed from relationship issues and so the stats and facts here relate specifically to one-to-one relationships.

According to information on relationships sourced from https://review42.com/uk the average relationship only lasts 2 years and 9 months and the younger the couple, the shorter the relationship.

Steve's first two marriages happened before he was barely 20, my first marriage was when I was 18. Nowadays the average marrying age in the UK is 29 for women and 31 for men, with 89% of couples living together before getting hitched for an average of 4.9 years.

The point here is that relationships break up a lot! The reasons are infinite however one of the latest statistics is that *54% of people said that social media played a big part in their break-up*.

According to https://www.mcleanhospital.org/ in their article 'The Social Dilemma: Social Media and Your Mental Health' (sourced 22/10/2021), "using social media can cause anxiety, depression, and other health challenges."

People use social media to "boost self-esteem and feel a sense of belonging in their social circles, people post content with the hope of receiving positive feedback."

No wonder it becomes addictive. But what happens when the feedback is negative, when people make hurtful comments, post information that is untrue or damning? This is the dark side of social media, and it is this dark side that has contributed to the break-up statistics highlighted above.

Current Thinking & Making Changes

Relationship issues, break-ups, domestic abuse,

mental abuse, peer pressure, work pressures. All these contribute to poor mental health and can, as in our cases, lead to a dependency on food that makes us feel better and more able cope with those difficult situations.

 https://www.iser.essex.ac.uk/ published an article on 8th February 2016 called *'Is there a link between obesity and mental health'*.

The article talks about research into 'Adiposity', the state of being obese, and its relationship with poor mental health in middle age. The highest association with mental health was found in the age group 30s to 50s.

It also concluded that; "social isolation potentially experienced by people who are obese may be greater at younger than older ages."

There was uncertainty in the findings about whether people with disease develop poor mental health and obesity or that obesity causes poor mental health and disease or that poor mental health causes disease and obesity however, the recommendation was that clinicians should consider the relationship between the two, particularly in people between 30 and 60.

 You can read the full paper: *Association of Adiposity and Mental Health Functioning across the Lifespan: Findings from Understanding Society (The UK Household Longitudinal Study)* here: http://journals.plos.org/plosone/article?id=10.1371/journal.pone.0148561

A final word about making changes in this chapter on the impact of relationships on obesity.

One of the key proven factors in becoming obese is depression. Relationship issues and break-ups can be a key factor in depression.

We feel bad, we want to feel better. Some people drink, in extreme cases people resort to drugs but for Steve and I and many of you, we eat, nice food, tasty food, food that makes us feel loved and happy.

What needs to change is our attitude. Food, long term is not going to make us feel better, look better, live longer or solve our problems. But food itself is not the enemy, it does not make us eat it, it does not make us fat on purpose, we do that to ourselves.

What is needed, in our opinion, is better support for people with depression, mental health issues and addiction, to help them to get the tools they need to overcome their challenges in a way that is not dependent on food, alcohol or drugs.

How Are Your Relationships Right Now?

Do you think that your relationship with food becomes self-destructive when your relationships go wrong? In the following section answer the questions to increase your self-awareness around your relationships and how they might be impacting on your weight.

Questions & Answers:

Are you in a happy relationship right now and if so, what do you consider to be 'happy'?

_____

_____

_____

Do you have issues that you have brought with you from one relationship to another?

_____

_____

_____

If you argue with a partner, what do you do afterwards to make yourself feel better?

_____

_____

_____

How did your relationship with your parents affect your attitude towards food?

_____

_____

_____

If you have had a breakup in the past, did you gain weight or lose weight, in the short term and long term?

_____

_____

_____

In a relationship, does your partner compliment you and make you feel good or critisise you?

_____

_____

_____

Are you slimmer when you are single or when you are in a relationship?

_____

_____

_____

Do any of your answers to the above questions raise any concerns for you? Do you need support in tackling relationship issues in order to maintain good mental health? If so, please seek professional support to address any issues you may have.

What Have You Learned About Yourself?

Thoughts Capture:

_____
_____
_____
_____
_____
_____
_____
_____
_____
_____
_____
_____
_____
_____
_____
_____
_____
_____
_____
_____
_____
_____

_____

_____

_____

_____

_____

_____

_____

_____

_____

_____

_____

_____

_____

What changes are you going to make in your life based on what you have learned?

Action Planner:

Changes I need to make in my life:

1. _____
   _____
   _____
2. _____
   _____
3. _____
   _____
4. _____
   _____

The Must Be More to Life Than This . . . ?

The Must Be More to Life Than This . . . ?

4: Health, Physical and Mental – cause or symptom?

Steve's Story – Health / Ill Health

My mental health problems, as we have seen from my story so far, have come mainly from my early childhood trauma and the loss of relationships throughout my life.

As a young man I was physically fit and healthy although I drank too much. My weight problems only really began after the breakdown of my marriage and loss of my mother in 2002, when I was 34 years old.

As an overweight man my mental health has declined further as I have battled physical and mental abuse. I am regularly mocked and abused because of my weight. From name calling to being spat on ...it is horrible, and most people don't realise how much it hurts. Unless you've been through it yourself, people don't understand the impact of this kind of discrimination.

I'm afraid to leave my home now, for fear of the abuse, made very much worse by the notoriety I gained after my TV appearances in 2015. I just want people to leave me alone and let me focus on getting better and helping other people.

Mental health issues first, leading to drink and food addiction, resulting in weight gain, followed by abuse, leading to declining mental health and continued addiction and physical health issues.

Even my experience of getting help has often been demoralising and embarrassing.

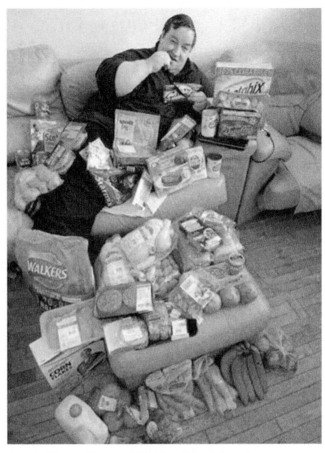

Image: Barry Gomer / Sunday People

After suffering a heart attack, a time when I was afraid of what was going to happen to me, when I should have been taken care of, I found myself having to wait for treatment because there were no beds strong enough to support me.

Much of my experience with doctors and hospitals has left me feeling like some staff are against me. There is a stigma that because of my weight I'm no good. There aren't chairs available that I can sit on in the doctor's waiting room or the right sized beds available in the hospital. There can be little understanding of the issues that people with obesity regularly face.

My mission now is to help others suffering from the issues arising from living with obesity, to try to remove the stigma and gain understanding of what is, in essence, a side effect of poor mental heath, stress, anxiety and trauma.

I know what I want to do. My dream job is to help people and tell them I've been there. I know lots of people like me.

Stigma can be a problem about getting jobs or just walking down the road and being spat at called fat fuck or fat bastard. One time being beaten, kicked, even pissed on. It was horrible people can be so cruel.

After hitting my top weight of 35 stone I felt like I was trapped in my own body, I hadn't left home for weeks. Even the thought of getting in the car was too much for me. I had given up and was waiting to die because I don't know what to do."

Even if I could make it out of the flat I just can't take the abuse from strangers in the street.

People call me a fat bastard, they tell me to stop eating all the pies and get another job, it makes me scared to leave the flat.

Getting bigger is my fault because I'm the one eating all the food. But getting so many insults makes me eat even more.

There's always a story behind a weight problem, you don't know what people like me are going through.

So far I have always resisted having a gastric band, because I doesn't believe in them, but now I think it might be time. I'm not sure that there is any other option for me.

I'm in pain the minute I try to get out my front door, my heart beats faster and I get out of breath. I feel shattered, so leaving the flat isn't an option.

I have had three strokes, I take medication following my heart attack, I'm on anti-depressants and I need two carers to come in daily to wash and dress me.

Mental health issues first, leading to drink and food addiction, resulting in weight gain, followed by abuse, leading to declining mental health and continued addiction and physical health issues.

I live in a continual cycle of physical and mental ill health.

Obesity As a Disease

Why would anyone consciously choose to become obese?

Obesity is soul destroying, it takes away your health, your confidence, your dignity, and in extreme cases, your will to live.

It reduces your chances of finding work, getting a promotion, being taken seriously by your peers and by its nature, makes everything you do harder and more tiring.

Obesity is a disease that is caused by eating more than the body needs to maintain a healthy function. The excess consumed is stored in the body as fat and increases until we either begin to eat less than we need to maintain that weight; or exercise more to burn up the calories stored, or both.

The question is, what causes someone to eat more than is necessary to maintain a healthy, functioning body?

Here are a few reasons why we start to overeat:

- It makes us feel better
- We like the taste and want more
- Chemicals in certain foods trigger our brains to want more of it
- Childhood conditioning, 'clear your plate or you won't get any pudding'.
- Dessert is a reward
- It is often the center of social occasions
- It comforts us when we feel down

So, the obesity starts to creep up on us. Well, you might ask, why don't people just stop overeating when they realise they are putting on weight?

This is where it gets complicated. I believe that there is a sort of tipping point. A place in time and space when you realise that you are overweight (it can take a while to be recognised because we generally don't want to acknowledge it).

When you get to that point you may have the emotional strength to say, 'enough is enough, let's sort this', I hope you do. In people who continue to gain weight it is because when we reach the tipping point, we:

- Hate ourselves for letting ourselves get to this point

- Think that we should be punished for getting to this point

- Believe we are not worth helping

- Have become addicted to the 'high' we get from sugar and high fat foods

- Feel so miserable about being overweight that we eat to make ourselves feel better

Ok, to a rational person this might seem like crazy thinking but at that tipping point, we are not always rational. Add to that the fact that overeating / food addiction is often a result of mental health issues such as depression, trauma, self-hate etc. then you might be able to begin to understand that our freedom to make rational choices just isn't there when we need it.

So, we continue to overeat, hate ourselves more, feel tired and unhappy, eat more to make ourselves feel better, hate ourselves more, continue to feel tired and unhappy, eat more to make ourselves feel better, hate ourselves more . . . and so it continues until one day, as in Steve's case, it all becomes just too much and we don't want to live anymore.

Stats & Facts

According to the NHS Health Survey for England 2019: 27% of men and 29% of women were obese. Around two thirds of adults were overweight or obese, this was more prevalent among men (68%) than women (60%).

The risk of diabetes in obese adults was 9% higher than in adults of a normal healthy weight.

The Priory Group state that, "It has become increasingly clear that obesity may also be a side effect of medications used to manage mental health issues. Increased appetite or overwhelming lethargy can both contribute to undesired weight gain and the associated long-term consequences."

They also quote the statistic that, "people who were obese had a 55% increased risk of developing depression over time, whereas people experiencing depression had a 58% increased risk of becoming obese. "

 (https://www.priorygroup.com/blog/the-relationship-between-mental-health-and-obesity)

The charity MIND included a graphic in their 2016 publication, 'Obesity and Mental Health' (https://mindcharity.co.uk/wp-content/uploads/2016/03/Obesity-and-Mental-Health.pdf) which clearly demonstrates the link between obesity and common mental health disorders.

Model for the mediator/moderator relationship between obesity and common mental health disorders:

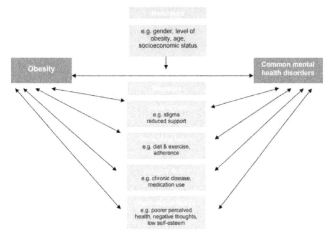

Source: Adapted from Markowitz et al. 2008 and Napolitano et al. 2008[4,5]

Current Thinking & Making Changes

I am an intelligent, successful businesswoman with a loving family and a life I love. I am also morbidly obese. I am not stupid, I did not consciously choose to be fat, it crept up on me over many years as a result of eating to make myself feel better, to compensate when things were going badly.

I passed the tipping point into self-loathing and have been on a constant battle to regain a normal weight and good mental and physical health ever since.

I have now developed a program to help others like me, middle aged women wanting to live a healthier, happier life, with confidence and positivity. It is called '**Think Mood Not Food'** and is all about dealing with the emotions associated with overeating.

The program gives you tools to help you become much more self-aware, in relation to both your failures and successes. We give you a methodology for weight loss that does not include dieting, calorie counting or any of those things which take so much effort and thought.

In the first two months of following the program I lost over a stone, and in those 2 months I went on holiday to Italy, ate out often, never gave up anything I love to eat or drink and didn't feel deprived even once.

We deal with what makes us overeat and how to change that. Focus on Mood, not Food.

This is how I am successfully battling my weight demons and you can have it too. Just go to the following web address to find out more and register:

https://alibagleycoach.samcart.com/products/mood-not-food

We have already talked about government initiatives to reduce sugar and promote healthy eating, but this misses the point. *It's not what we eat that needs to be addressed, it's why we eat it.*

Until more is done to address the mental health issues that lead to obesity it will always be there. Diets don't work, reducing sugar and fats in foods doesn't work, banning anything 'fattening' is ridiculous and totally impractical.

Education and understanding is what is needed. Tolerance and acceptance of what obese people are going through, not hate and abuse.

What Is Your Current State of Health?

 Questions and Answers

Are you happy?

_____

_____

_____

Do you take medication for any mental health issues?

_____

_____

_____

Do you have any physical health issues that have resulted in depression or other mental health issues?

_____

_____

_____

Are you a healthy weight and if not how much extra weight are you carrying?

_____

_____

_____

Would you say that you are at or past the tipping point to be able to deal rationally you're your weight issue?

_____

_____

_____

_____

Have you experienced physical health issues as a result of a weight problem / obesity?

_____

_____

_____

Have you experienced weight issues as a result of a physical health problem?

_____

_____

_____

Are you currently trying to improve your overall physical and mental health and wellbeing or is it all too overwhelming for you?

_____

_____

_____

_____

What Have You Learned About Yourself?

Thoughts Capture:

_____

_____

_____

_____

The Must Be More to Life Than This . . . ?

What changes are you going to make in your life based on what you have learned?

Action Planner:

Changes I need to make in my life:

1. _____
_____
_____
_____

2. _____
_____
_____

3. _____
_____
_____

4. _____
_____
_____
_____

The Must Be More to Life Than This . . . ?

5: Try, try and try again

Steve's Story – Triumphs & Failures

My mental health issues resulted in years of addiction. Firstly to alcohol as a teenager, and then to food, the addiction that led to me becoming morbidly obese and entering a vicious cycle of eat to feel better, gain weight, self-loathing, eat to feel better.

I have also manifested other classic symptoms of depression including self-harm, suicide attempts, and an inability to cope with failed relationships.

During my six marriages I have found maintaining healthy, loving relationships a challenge and even now, with wife Michelle, although I am happy there have been difficult times.

In 2015 I featured on Channel 5s "Too Fat To Work" programme with Michelle. I decided to take part after being convinced it would be a positive experience, highlighting the problems associated with the stigma of obesity in the UK.

Michelle and I both committed to the programme and between us we lost a great deal of weight but the programme that aired was not what I had expected. Instead, I felt that it portrayed me as lazy and stupid, and I was denounced in the media as 'Britain's fattest scrounger'.

Boot camp was hard, waking at 5am every day to go to the gym. It was hard going but I had to do it, the weight was killing me. We were separated from friends and family for 6 months and had to live in a caravan, but we did it to try to help people see that we wanted to get fit and get jobs

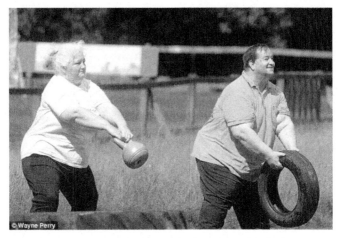

The boot camp saved my life but the media attention and hate that came afterwards drove me to try and kill myself by jumping off a bridge. I failed and I was sectioned for 72 hours, receiving the help and support I needed but still continuing to self-harm and go deeper into depression when I got home.

I was afraid to leave my flat because of the attacks, couldn't even answer the phone, and ended up in a financial mess as the programme and my representatives had taken everything we had.

It wasn't until a year later, in 2016 that I realised and accepted that I had an eating disorder and addiction, and it was actually ok to admit to and discuss my problems.

Appearances on Good Morning Britain followed and being able to talk about my issues in public was a real relief for me.

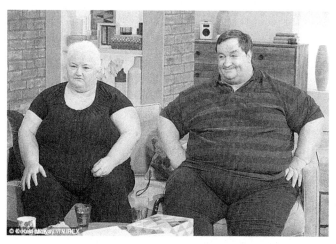

However, my appearances on the Jeremy Kyle show again sent me into depression. My experience was that I had been 'set up' by the production team in order to sensationalise my story and even made to look as if I had been having an affair, which I hadn't.

I was finally diagnosed with Borderline Personality Disorder, I sought help and now I talk openly and honestly about my condition to help others. I am also now an advocate of child obesity awareness and men's mental illness.

With borderline personality disorder (BPD), one minute I am on high the next I could cry, I am sad, depressed its horrible, I even lost a lot of friends over having this.

I feel that I am 2 people in one body, it's strange and it's the not knowing what's going to happen next, or my change of attitude towards people. Sometimes I have to say sorry to people that I hurt or am not nice to.

I think with me the illness has definitely not helped

me; I have hurt people. It makes me feel so sad that I have done this to many people who I love and respect, its soul destroying.

But I am a survivor. I may have seemingly insurmountable problems to overcome as a result of my obesity and mental health issues but I am determined to dedicate the time and energy I have to helping others through my work with the stroke community, my podcast and as an ambassador for mental health.

Why We Fail in Our Battle Against Obesity

If losing weight was easy no one would be fat. If gaining weight was difficult, there would be far less obesity.

In her article, 'Why Diets Don't Work', Maureen Moerbeck of **Nutritionist Resource** states that, "It's not surprising that we are seduced into dieting. We live in a society that praises thinness in women and muscularity in men, and these traits are portrayed as something to be desired – a sign of confidence, health, and achievement. Therefore, if we do not fit into this mould, we can be made to feel unhealthy, lazy and "less than".

Straight away we feel 'failure' in that we have been unable to meet societal norms and so we look for a solution, a quick fix, to get us beck to being 'acceptable'. So we decide to 'go on a diet'.

Of course, the multi-billion-pound diet industry is so successful exactly because diets don't work. They depend on repeat custom and to get that, people have to 'fail' to lose the weight they want to, or at least regain it as soon as they stop dieting.

And so begins the cycle of yoyo dieting, experienced by so many. In my lifetime I would estimate that I have probably lost over 50 stone on diets, and that I have regained at least 60!

Stats & Facts

In her article Maureen also states that, "The yo-yoing in weight that happens after going on diet after diet can be more damaging to our physical health than maintaining a higher weight i.e. not dieting in the first place. Not to mention, there are detrimental psychological and emotional effects of being on a diet and feeling you are "failing"."

Furthermore, constant dieting has been proven to actually slow down your metabolic rate, the speed at which your body processes the calories it ingests. When your metabolism slows down your body tries even harder to conserve energy and stores it in the form of fat.

Statistically, approximately 68% of men and 58% of women in the UK are classed as overweight.

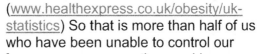 (www.healthexpress.co.uk/obesity/uk-statistics) So that is more than half of us who have been unable to control our weight, for one reason or another, and have therefore 'failed' to conform to the accepted norm of a healthy slim body. That's a lot of 'failure' to deal with.

Steve is an extreme example of someone who's eating habits have gone out of control, over a long period of time, and who now feels that his only option is gastric band surgery.

We know that dealing with the cause of overeating is key. It's not what we eat, but why we eat it that needs to be addressed. Diets only deal with the 'what' we eat. More education and help is needed to help us to understand the 'why' we eat it.

In the next section answer the questions and think about what triggers your inability to control your weight gain. Look back again at your Emotional Map for insight into why you 'fail' and 'succeed'.

What Triggers Your Downfall?

Questions and Answers

How many times have you been on a diet in the last 5 years?

_____

_____

_____

Did those diets fully address why you overate or just how to change your eating habits?

_____

_____

_____

What do you think are the situations or events that trigger you to overeat?

1._____

2._____

3._____

4._____

5._____

6._____

7._____

8._____

9._____

10._____

How long, on average, do you stick to a diet for?

_____

_____

_____

What usually makes you stop following a diet?

_____

_____

_____

What help / support do you really think you need in order to get to and maintain a healthy weight?

_____

_____

_____

_____

_____

_____

_____

_____

_____

What Have You Learned About Yourself?

Thoughts Capture:

_____

_____

_____

_____

_____

_____

_____

_____

The Must Be More to Life Than This . . . ?

What changes are you going to make in your life based on what you have learned?

Action Planner:

Changes I need to make in my life:

1. _____
   _____
   _____
   _____
2. _____
   _____
3. _____
   _____
4. _____
   _____
   _____

The Must Be More to Life Than This . . . ?

The Must Be More to Life Than This . . . ?

6: Vilification – why do people act the way they do?

Steve's Story – Vilification on a Massive Scale

For most of us, hopefully, nastiness directed our way is fairly uncommon. I like to believe that most people are basically decent and kind to one another.

During the times I have been attacked, verbally or physically in my life I haven't been in any real immediate danger and the occurrences have mostly been in private.

Steve, on the other hand, has been subjected to extreme nastiness and all in the public eye.

He has appeared on several TV shows in the last few years. These include This Morning, The Jeremy Kyle show, and Channel 5s 'Too Fat To Work'.

Heres how he tells it . . .

As an overweight man unable to work because of my obesity and living in virtual isolation in my small flat with Michelle I was attracted to the idea of being on TV.

I had several appearances on the Jeremy Kyle show but the show almost ended my marriage with a staged affair and a constant effort by the producers to 'wind me up' before I went on air.

The producers staged the affair with myself and Melissa. She wanted to go on the show anyway but the story about the affair is fake.

The stint on Channel 5s 'Too Fat to Work'

programme started out well. We both hoped that this would help us to lose weight and get our lives back on track, and we did both lose a lot of weight over the time we were in the boot camp, 17 stone between us over the six months.

However, after the show was aired, the reaction from the press and the public nearly drove me to suicide.

Labelled as 'Britain's Fattest Scrounger', I found myself being attacked by the media as a lazy benefits scrounger who had no intention of working and expecting the government to support me.

The truth of the matter is that I was trying really hard to get slimmer and fitter. I had worked all my life up to the point where I became physically unable to do so. Not highly educated, but not stupid either, the kind of work I could do was mostly manual, like my jobs as a club bouncer and a window cleaner. I want to work, I just can't.

I lost a lot of weight and then I put some weight back on again because I relapsed... I was so ashamed that I tried to actually kill myself.

The trouble is, when you are being called scrounger and a lot of things going in your head and about life, all of a sudden mentally... it could happen to anyone, depression.

I was dealing with the grief of us losing our baby, not having a job, and we were living in a terrible flat that was really damp, and I had a lot of family issues. I went to Tamar Bridge and I tried to jump off it. I did that twice.

Fortunately, both times Michelle alerted the police and they came and arrested me under the Mental

Health Act. She was very upset about it.

I also applied for Big Brother USA, although I thought that I was applying for the UK version. Unfortunately, I didn't have a passport so couldn't make the audition as I had hoped to try and put my side of things out to the public.

What I am doing now is investing my time in supporting other stroke victims and trying to create more discussion and visibility around the profound effect of poor mental health on obesity.

A RAY OF HOPE

Too often I've hidden inside me,

Safe inside, in my shell, no-one near.

Ashamed of myself for my failures,

Unable to laugh or to cheer.

I see others out there in the sunlight,

Smiling and happy and free.

I stay in the darkness alone here,

Unwilling to live and be me.

What if they say that I'm ugly,

What if they laugh at my shape.

How can I let others judge me,

What if I only find hate.

But if I stay hidden forever
My life will be wasted and gone.
Should I let what they might say about me,
Imprison me here for so long.

I'm stronger than that and I know it,
No more hiding and crying and loss.
I'm making my way to the sunlight,
I'm going to show them who's boss.

The time has come to be brave now,
To stand up and be who I am.
Get out there and live life completely,
To be the best that I can.

So haters stand back cos I'm coming,
I don't care what anyone says.
I'm finally going to beat this,
And be happy the rest of my days.

A poem by Ali Bagley

Why Are People So Nasty?

First of all, let me state this very clearly:

When people are nasty to you or about you, it is not about you, it is about them

Steve has been spat at in the street and called horrible names. It's not his fault, he didn't ask for that treatment, his being obese did not make those people behave in the way they did.

People are nasty for many reasons, in my experience, mostly because of their own fears and inadequacies. The press are deliberately nasty to sell papers and attract viewers. The trick is to not allow those people and their behaviours to have an impact on how you feel about yourself.

Some people are very sly in their nastiness, undermining and belittling you in an attempt to gain control over you. This was what happened to me in my first marriage. Constant little jibes and put downs that I allowed to erode my confidence and self-esteem.

My husband was terrified that I would leave him so behaved this way so that I would lose my will. I was stronger than that and was able to leave but I still carry the mental scars.

Others are more direct and vocal, the boss showing you up in a meeting to make himself look better or pass the blame onto you, the 'friend' who tells publicly you that you need to lose weight or that your breath smells, not to help you but to make you feel bad.

These people have a need to be seen as the best. The top of the tree, the achievers, the most popular. They act this way in order to make themselves out to be better than you.

Then there are the bullies. The small-minded individuals who feel the need to stamp their authority by attacking you either physically or verbally.

Bullies can do enormous damage to our self-esteem and mental wellbeing. Remember, they are the ones with the problem, not you. Feel sorry for them, pity them, it will help you to control their impact on you.

Stats & Facts

According to the Trade Union Congress in the UK about a third of people are bullied at work and women are more likely to be targeted. In nearly ¾ of cases bullying is carried out by a manager. And that is just the numbers we know about.

The office for National Statistics says that around 1 in 5 children between the ages of 10 and 15 are bullied and that in fact almost three quarters of children had experienced bullying in some form during their school years.

The rise of the smart phone has been widely blamed for these shocking figures. Online bullying can be done anonymously at the same time as being very public. The damage it causes ranges from upset right through to documented cases of suicide.

According to the CIPD (The professional body for HR and people development - https://www.cipd.co.uk/) harassment and bullying may be against one or more people and may involve single or repeated incidents across a wide spectrum of behaviour, ranging from extreme forms of intimidation, such as physical violence, to more subtle forms such as ignoring someone. It can occur without witnesses, in face-to-face interactions, as well as online. Examples include:

- Unwanted physical contact.

- Unwelcome remarks about a person's age, dress, appearance, race or marital status, jokes at personal expense, offensive language, gossip, slander, sectarian songs and letters.

- Posters, graffiti, obscene gestures, flags, bunting and emblems.

- Isolation or non-cooperation and exclusion from social activities.

- Coercion for sexual favours.

- Pressure to participate in political/religious groups.

- Personal intrusion from pestering, spying and stalking.

- Failure to safeguard confidential information

- Shouting and bawling.

- Setting impossible deadlines.

- Persistent unwarranted criticism.

- Personal insults.

Everything that Steve has experienced, the spitting, the name calling, the kicking, all these come under the term bullying and are totally unacceptable.

The Impact of Hateful Behaviour on Others

Bullying is another term for hateful behaviour.

There is a whole other book on why people bully others but right now we are looking at the effect their bullying has on us and how it impacts on our weight problem specifically.

Once again, we have the chicken and egg scenario, do people taunt us and attack us because we are obese or are we obese as a result of taunting and attacks in our past?

Possibly both in my case, and in Steve's. As a child he was bullied in school because he smelled of the fish his Dad worked with, "when I was with the family living on the Barbican my Mum and Dad was working in a crab factory. I used to go to school smelling of fish and it was horrible. I was bullied and hated being at school, a few times they spit in my food and pushed my head down the toilet. Life was horrible."

Can you imagine how the young Steve felt during those attacks, all because he smelled of fish. In the end he became pretty much a loner, preferring to stay out of the way of other children.

In later life, Steve was afraid to go out of his front door; regularly facing physical and verbal abuse when he walked down the street, returning him to the fear and hurt of his childhood bullying, and which left him feeling suicidal.

Stephen says, "I am regularly mocked and abused because of my weight. From name calling to being spat on ...it is horrible, and most people don't realise how much it hurts. Unless you've been through it yourself, people don't understand the impact of this kind of discrimination."

He says, "When I was young I was always a loner, I liked my own company for some reason even though I went to youth club and started a football team up."

"Do you get the feeling when you are out that people are looking at you and when you got a pasty or something to eat, they stare they walk off and you can hear the words 'he's big rolly polly, Telly Tubby etc. You feel horrible then. All you want to do is hurry home and shut the door and cry. We do live in a world of stigma and hate."

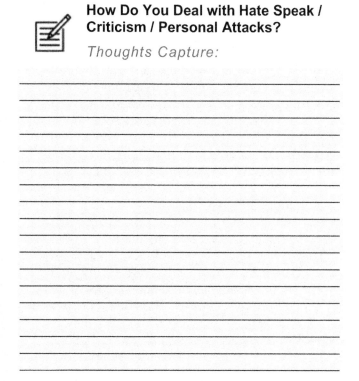

How Do You Deal with Hate Speak / Criticism / Personal Attacks?

Thoughts Capture:

 What Personally Can You Change to Make Things Better?

Hints, Tips & Ideas

1. Be mindful of the feelings of others.
2. Be kind whenever you can
3. Stand up for others who are being bullied
4. Develop your own self-confidence in order to withstand bullying against you
5. Help others to build their self-confidence
6. Do not tolerate discrimination of any kind
7. Think twice before you speak, think twice before you react, think twice before you let others bring you down
8. Remember that bullies are usually sad unhappy people and pity them
9. No-one has the power to make you feel bad, but you have the power to stop them
10. There will always be people worse off than you. Remember that when you feel sorry for yourself
11. Don't give up, you are unique and special and you have a right to be happy

The Must Be More to Life Than This . . . ?

The Must Be More to Life Than This . . . ?

7 Moving forward with hope

Steve's Story - Changes

The thing that most impresses me about Steve is his desire to help others even though he still needs so much help himself.

He not only has hope for his future, he helps others to find that hope too.

Here Steve tells us what he is up to right now . . .

Although I still need help to wash and dress every day and my mobility is very limited, I am not only running the local Exmouth Stroke Survivors Club, I am also the host and creator of an award winning podcast that I set up to help people to share their stories about coping whilst living a life with anxiety and depression.

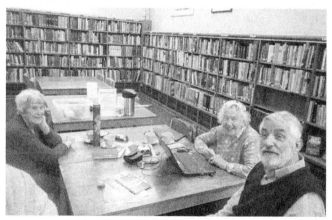

The original Exmouth Stroke Survivors Club

The Exmouth Stroke Survivors Club is a community group for people who have had a stroke to share experiences and make friends - and their family members and carers are welcome too.

I am the leader of the club having taken over after the previous leader and founder, Len, was unable to continue due to health issues.

We think Len deserves a knighthood! He needs a gold medal for what he's been through.

The club has grown since its inception in 2009 and now meets in Exmouth Library on Wednesday mornings from 10am-12pm. All are welcome, including family and carers

We want people to come along and get the help they deserve. If we can help just one person, we'll have done our job.

We've had people from Budleigh, Exeter, Paignton, Cornwall, join us. It's not just for stroke patients, it's for their families too.

The door's always open. There's 24-hour support for all the members. If someone came up to me and said, 'I don't feel well', we'll get in touch with a doctor and get help straight away.

We can do music, which is good for strokes - people can sing after a stroke (despite not being able to talk). If anybody's got some musical instruments to donate, we'd be very grateful. We go on trips, go to garden centers; and we play darts, draughts and dominoes.

 If you would like to join, please email me at: exmouth.stroke.survivors.club@gmail.com or visit:
https://www.exmouthstrokesurvivorsclub.com/

I am also campaigning against the opening of new fast-food outlets where I live in Plymouth. In fact I once chained myself to a fence outside of a new proposed fried chicken restaurant to try to stop it opening.

I think that councils should put tighter controls on takeaways opening in certain areas of towns and cities. The cheap and easy availabilities of takeaways in this area have contributed to my obesity, and I have campaigned against new branches of certain takeaways and fast-food outlets from opening in parts of Plymouth. There are 23 fast-food businesses on Victoria Street near my home, almost double the number that existed five years ago and that is way too many.

Whilst I know I can't stop them I thinks that there should be some kind of limit on how many can operate in one area.

And then there is the Podcast, but more about that in the next chapter.

Is There Hope?

There is always hope, always.

For years Steve was afraid to leave his flat for fear of judgement and was so desperate that he tried to take his own life, on more than one occasion.

Now look at what he is achieving.

For years I had no confidence and hated how I looked, and now I am running a successful business and working as the Director of an International Coaching Platform as well as becoming a bestselling author.

If Steve and I can turn our lives around and be successful, then you can too.

Why don't you go back to your emotional map, that you developed after reading Chapter 1, and run through all the notes you have made on what you have learned.

Using all of that information, why not draw a new map, using the same emotional geography methodology and this time drawing your future. Your dreams and goals. When do you want to achieve them, how are you going to do it, how will you overcome obstacles?

Make a plan for your future success. Don't let anyone tell you that you can't do it, you can.

Stats & Facts

Statistics on hope are hard to find, after all hope is a very subjective emotion and means different things to different people, so is not easy to measure.

However, there is a link between hope and its impact on health and happiness.

In an article by Paula Davis J.D. M.A.P.P entitled **5 Ways Hope Impacts Health and Happiness** (5 ways the science of hope influences the way you work and life) 2013, https://www.psychologytoday.com/us/blog/pressure-proof/201303/5-ways-hope-impacts-health-happiness we can see that employees with higher hope levels are absent from work less often, that hopeful salespeople do better than those less hopeful, that working towards life goals is one of the key elements of hope and it makes you happy, that hopeful people feel less pain in illness than others and that as long as you have hope you are more likely to live longer.

Here is the dictionary definition of hope:

NOUN

1. a feeling of expectation and desire for a particular thing to happen.

   "he looked through her belongings in the hope of coming across some information"

   synonyms:

   aspiration · desire · wish · expectation · ambition · aim · plan · dream · daydream · pipe dream · longing · yearning · craving · hankering

2. archaic

   a feeling of trust.

   "our private friendship, upon hope and affiance whereof, I presume to be your petitioner"

VERB

1. want something to happen or be the case.

   "he's hoping for an offer of compensation"

   synonyms:

   expect · anticipate · look for · wait for · be hopeful of · pin one's hopes on · want · wish for · dream of · hope against hope for

Why Make Changes At All?

Well honestly, you don't have to. You can continue just as you are if you want to. Do you want to?

Things change around us all the time and if we don't change and adapt along with them then we are in danger of being left behind.

I love this saying from Heraclitus, an ancient Greek philosopher:

"You cannot step into the same river twice, for other waters are continually flowing on."

This idea that the water and life within a river are always changing, even if the river looks the same, can be applied to life in general. People are never the same, changing always from our day-to-day experiences, and in society.

Steve and I both know that we need to change our attitude and approach to eating and our food addictions in order to get healthy and feel better about ourselves and our lives.

We hope, with this book, that we have encouraged you to gain a better understanding of how we became obese, of your relationship with food and your attitude towards obesity, and if necessary, to make changes to be more tolerant and supportive, of others as well as of yourself.

You can choose to stay just as you are, and that if ok. Or you can strive every day to be a better person, for yourself and for others.

What Do You Want to Change About Your Life?

Goals & Targets

I want to . . .

1. _____
   _____
   _____

2. _____
   _____
   _____

3. _____
   _____
   _____

4. _____
   _____
   _____

5. _____
   _____
   _____

6. _____
   _____
   _____

7. _____
   _____
   _____

Creating an Action Plan that is SMART

Action Plan

SMART stands for **S**pecific, **M**easurable, **A**chievable, **R**elevant, and **T**ime-bound

As you create your new map for your future goals and aspirations and using your list of your goals and targets, use the table below to detail how you are going to do it, why you are going to do it and how it will benefit you, remembering all the time to keep those goals SMART.

1. Goal / Target

_____

How

_____

Why

_____

Benefit

_____

_____

2. Goal / Target

_____

How

_____

Why

_____

Benefit

_____

_____

_____

3. Goal / Target

_____

How

_____

Why

_____

Benefit

_____

_____

4. Goal / Target

_____

How

_____

Why

_____

Benefit

_____

_____

5. Goal / Target

_____

How

_____

Why

_____

Benefit

_____

_____

6. Goal / Target

_____

How

_____

Why

_____

Benefit

_____

_____

_____

7. Goal / Target

_____

How

_____

Why

_____

Benefit

_____

_____

_____

8 The Podcast – Steve making a difference in the world

Ali's Interview with Steve

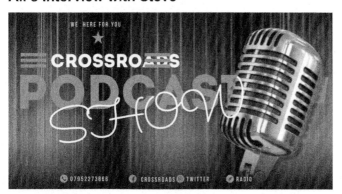

Steve, What is The Podcast?

In July 2020 I was bored with just staying at home and watching the TV. With Covid no-one was going out and I knew I wasn't the only one sat at home bored.

So, one day, out of the blue I had an idea to start a podcast and a radio station. I thought it would be a great thing to do to help people connect with each other and maybe share their thoughts and problems about depression and anxiety.

So how did you start?

Well first I needed to come up with a name and I decided to go with Crossroads podcast because we were all at a crossroads right then.

Was it difficult to get started?

Not really, I just had to set it up on Streamyard and find people to interview and things to talk about. I did the first show from my bedroom.

How did you feel that first time?

Well I got myself ready, had a shave and a shower and then I went live. I was really nervous but I actually did two shows that day.

How was it received?

It was slow at first but after a while loads of people were asking to come on and I was doing sometimes several broadcasts a day. Audience numbers were growing and people were leaving great reviews.

Who comes on as guests?

We have had all sorts, sometimes talking about anxiety and depression but lots of other things too. I even had a Buddhist Monk on once.

How many listeners do you have now?

Today we have more than 52,000 listeners, including football stars and other people from all walks of life.

What do you want to achieve with the Podcasts Steve?

Life is hard for everybody in one way or another. I hope that through the podcast people will feel less alone with their problems, maybe get good advice and learn something and most of all to help people to understand that depression and anxiety can happen to anyone, but we can get through it with support and kindness.

Especially with Covid and so many people feeling alone and unhappy.

What Are You Most Proud Of and Why?

I am proud that so many people listen and they say such nice things. I am also really proud of the fact that what we talk about on the show really helps people.

What Feedback Have You Had From Listeners?

Absolutely loads and nearly always very kind and supportive. Here are a few:

Excellent a real gem of podcasts. Susanne K

Steve was a great host! He asked amazing questions and kept the audience engaged. It was a very refreshing and positive environment and I felt very comfortable. I definitely recommend tuning into his show. You will not be disappointed! Brooklyn B

Steve Beer is a kind and sincere host at Crossroads Podcast Show who is passionate about serving others and providing positive and valuable insights and information to his audience. He's authentic about helping to make this world a better place for us all. Stacy B

I really enjoyed my first trip to your podcast Steve! Thank you for sharing your story and book plans alongside my own 😊 **I very much look forward to next time.** Lisa Maria C

I have just done my podcast with Steve - the first time I have been let loose to actually tell my story in full ..... Love the show and have been invited back ...... 😁. Lee C

I was invited to participate in Steve's podcast back in September and this was my first ever guest spot on a podcast ever.

It was great, the questions were good and allowed me to explain fully about how I work with businesses who want to raise money through finance, investment or crowdfunding. he number of people who saw this is astounding. I've had messages from all over the world as a follow on from appearing on this podcast. It was a brilliant way to market myself.

Thanks Steve and team x Nicola T

I loved chatting with Steve for the Crossroads Podcast and love the work he's doing. It's so important for people to have a safe space to share their story and where they feel they have a voice. He's a good listener and a great interviewer. Michele EH

Great interview with Steve on his Crossroads podcast show where we talked about all sorts from women and money, to property and to homelessness. Highly recommend Steve and his podcast show. Caitriona E

Steve, thank you for the opportunity it was a super experience and to know you are there helping people too. You created a relaxed atmosphere and are liked by many I am sure. See you next month! Highly recommended.😁 Jan M

Steve Beer is does an amazing show, and I love that he is doing this show to bring people together. . . Thank you for everything you do. Jake E

Wow Steve is an amazing man here to do so much good in the world. We really need to talk about mental resilience and be here to support each other, and Steve is so brave to stand up and do that! Very entertaining . . . and his show is epic - definitely go watch it for yourself. Michelle C

For a person from India, getting interviewed by Steve was a big event for me. I was very nervous. But Steve with his calm soothing manner put me at ease.

His questions touched on all the subjects I really wanted to talk about.

With his in depth probing I was able to put my point across. I found the experience amazing.

Thanks Steve for a lovely time. Shaista F

What's next For the Podcast?

Steve continues to broadcast most days and is always looking for new guests who have something to share with others.

 If you want to be a guest or just tune in go to:
https://www.facebook.com/crossroadspodcastuk/photos/a.136787411446535/391283965996877/

Thanks Steve, I have been a guest twice now and I can vouch for the fact that it is a great show and is really helping people to connect.

We even launched the book on the Podcast:

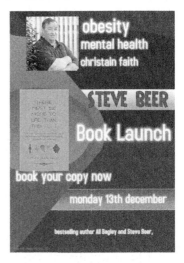

Stats & Facts

On average 6.5 million people in the UK listen to podcasts each week and of those 63% of listeners are men.

According to **the podcast host** (https://www.thepodcasthost.com/) There are 4,180,000 total podcasts registered, around the world. (podcastindex.org – September 2021)

However, the percentage of active podcasts has dropped from 59% in December 2020 to 34% in June 2021.

Maybe that is because we are all returning to more face-to-face interaction now.

The most popular podcast genres for men are sports, comedy and music. For women lifestyle, current affairs and wellbeing rank high.

Steve's Story

The podcast **is** Steve's story. He shares so much of himself, his fears, challenges and triumphs on there that instead of a story for this chapter I simply ask you to go and tune in.

 Details can be found here:

https://www.facebook.com/crossroadspodcastuk/photos/a.136787411446535/391283965996877/

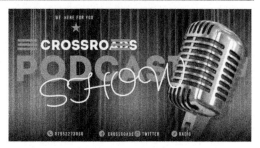

The Must Be More to Life Than This . . . ?

9: Finding the help you need

Steve's Story – Who He Is Helping Now

I want to help people. Yes, I have my own battles to fight with my weight and depression but even so, helping others helps me to put things into perspective and feel better about everything.

For the first time in my life I am doing things for other people in a way that makes me feel useful and needed and I am actually getting respect now, instead of abuse and hate all the time.

Just look at the reviews for my podcast. Plus, getting membership of a national obesity forum and being able to change people's views with this book and my campaigning has been fantastic.

On a more local scale I also enjoy the work I do with the stroke club and now I am on the council committee for housing locally in Exeter which is an honour and I hope to make a difference with my work there too.

For so many years I just sat in my flat, eating, feeling miserable, then getting heavier and feeling more miserable. Yes, I lost a load of weight on the 'Too Fat to Work' programme, but I regained it quickly because nothing I have done has ever really helped me to get to the bottom of my weight problem, the real reason why I got to where I am and how I can change it.

As Ali says, it's not what you eat, it's why you eat, and I need to do some work on that.

The question is, what help is available and how do I access that?

Michelle is 50 this year, I am 53, we should have years ahead of us to do the things we want to do.

What Help Is Out There For You?

Throughout this book we have highlighted the fact that obesity is a disease, usually a side effect of poor mental health and most definitely not a conscious choice we make.

If we fall over and break our leg we go to hospital and they fix it. If we have a cold we take ourselves off to bed until we feel better, if we get cancer then we get comprehensive treatment and support from the NHS.

If we get fat we get ridiculed or ignored and recovery from being fat i.e. losing weight, is something that we are expected to sort out for ourselves.

- Join a diet club (short term fix, long term problems)
- See you doctor (recommends a diet club!)
- Work out why you are fat (costly private counselling or a horrendously long wait on an NHS waiting list)
- Get a weight loss coach (good but pricey)
- Ask for gastric band surgery (costly private or long NHS waiting list)
- Get liposuction (short term fix, very expensive)
- Buy pills off the internet (please DO NOT

DO THIS, it might kill you)
- See a nutritionist to develop a healthy eating program for you (pricey and still not sorting the underlying problem)

In writing this book I started to research where we could get help to fix the underlying issue with obesity, i.e., why we get fat in the first place.

As an Emotional Geographer with my Mood Not Food Program I am changing my mindset first and that in turn has helped me to create new healthy living habits. And I say healthy living, not healthy eating because obesity is about lifestyle, not food by itself.

As my mother used to say, "nothing is fattening until you eat too much of it."

Looking at my emotional relationship with food through geo-emotional mapping, analysing my strengths, weaknesses and trigger points and then dealing with the issues that caused me to overeat in the first place has been the best thing I ever did in my journey towards a healthier life.

I know now the reasons why I got so fat. I also have the tools to lose the excess weight and live a healthier lifestyle. I am not dieting, I have simply changed my attitude towards food by understanding my mental health issues.

Stats & Facts

"Today, what we know is that when obesity and issues with mental health are found to co-exist, they can create a negative spiral effect for any individual. Each condition will continually aggravate the other, which in turn only creates a vicious cycle. This makes it difficult to determine which condition was present first, which also makes the overall situation worse." Merrill Littleberry, 2017 (https://www.obesityaction.org/community/article-library/obesity-and-mental-health-is-there-a-link/)

 According to MIND, the mental health charity (https://mindcharity.co.uk/wp-content/uploads/2016/03/Obesity-and-Mental-Health.pdf) in their publication, 'Obesity and mental health', the following issues are identified:

- Both obesity and common mental health disorders account for a significant proportion of the global burden of disease.
- There are bi-directional associations between mental health problems and obesity, with levels of obesity, gender, age and socioeconomic status being key risk factors.
- The mental health of women is more closely affected by overweight and obesity than that of men.
- There is strong evidence to suggest an association between obesity and poor mental health in teenagers and adults. This evidence is weaker for younger children.
- The relationships between actual body weight, self-perception of weight and weight stigmatisation are complex and this varies across cultures, age and ethnic groups.
- The perception of being obese appears to be more predictive of mental disorders than

actual obesity in both adults and children.

- Weight stigma increases vulnerability to depression, low self-esteem, poor body image, maladaptive eating behaviours and exercise avoidance.
- Intervention strategies should consider both the physical and mental health of patients. It has been recommended that care providers should monitor the weight of depressive patients and, similarly, in overweight or obese patients, mood should be monitored. This awareness could lead to prevention, early detection, and co-treatment for people at risk, ultimately reducing the burden of both conditions.
- There is an urgent need for evaluations of weight management interventions, both in terms of weight loss and psychological benefits.

Where Can You Find the Help You Need?

Here are the organisations that I have found online that offer services in relation to addressing the mental health issues related to obestity.

This list is not comprehensive but is a good started as you search for your solutions.

I am not recommending any diet clubs, programs or organisations unless their service is based in tackling the underlying causes of obesity.

1. **HOOP UK:** a unique group of passionate people, including professionals, with the common aim to make the changes needed

so that all children and adults struggling with obesity are given access to the services which are right for them.
http://hoopuk.org.uk/

2. **NHS Obesity site**: https://www.nhs.uk/conditions/obesity/ for information and guidance about obesity including the link to their social care and support guide. https://www.nhs.uk/conditions/social-care-and-support-guide/

3. **The National Centre for Eating Disorders**: information and professional training in the help & treatment of eating disorders. Eating disorders, such as compulsive overeating, binge eating, anorexia, bulimia, obesity, orthorexia & failed dieting. http://www.eating-disorders.org.uk/

4. **The National Obesity Forum**: a charity formed in 2000, with the remit of raising awareness of obesity in the UK and promoting the ways in which it can be addressed. This includes public-facing initiatives and the training of clinicians and healthcare professionals on how to identify and address weight management issues and obesity. http://www.nationalobesityforum.org.uk/

5. **MaleVoiceED**: a charity providing a platform to all males enabling the sharing of narrative around poor relationships with food and co-morbid conditions. MaleVoicED also shares the experiences of caregivers, friends and associates who have been affected by such poor food related relationships.

http://www.malevoiced.com/

6. **Overeaters Anonymous**: a fellowship of individuals who, through shared experience, strength and hope are recovering from compulsive overeating. Welcomes everyone who wants to stop eating compulsively.
http://www.oagb.org.uk/

7. **Weight Concern**: this charity is committed to developing and researching new treatments for obesity. It is also working to increase the availability of the successful treatments it has pioneered in the UK via self-help programmes, self-help support groups and family based childhood obesity treatment.
http://www.weightconcern.org.uk/

8. **Weight Matters**: the UKs leading therapy centre for weight, food, eating and health issues. This organisation provides online therapy and counselling in relation to eating behaviour and weight issues. This treatment is private and as such will incur a cost.
https://www.weightmatters.co.uk/

9. **Weight Wise:** An independent site, managed by the British Dietetic Association (BDA), with unbiased, easy-to-follow hints and tips - based on the latest evidence - to help you manage your weight for good. It will help you take a look at your current eating habits and physical activity levels, and offer a practical approach to setting your own goals for lifestyle change.
http://www.bdaweightwise.com/

10. **The British Nutrition Foundation**: Promotes the wellbeing of society through the impartial interpretation and effective

dissemination of scientifically based knowledge and advice on the relationship between diet, physical activity and health. http://www.nutrition.org.uk/

Fat v Fit

Being fat doesn't necessarily mean that you are unfit, being fit does not necessarily mean that you are slim.

The point here is that if you carry a lot of excess weight, you will probably feel more sluggish, unhappy and less fit than if you can maintain a healthy weight.

There are many organisations that can help you with your weight issues yes, but there is also stuff you can do for yourself, right now, for free, that is going to benefit you and help you move towards a more healthy weight and lifestyle. What is it?

JUST MOVE

Move a little more each day than you did yesterday. I'm not suggesting you start training for the London Marathon (but hey, why not if that's a SMART Goal for you). I am suggesting walking a little further, a little faster, maybe going swimming once a week, dust off those old exercise DVDs and have a go.

Little extra steps every day.

Re-Visit Your Action Plan

Action Plan

All the way through this book you have been able to create mini action plans to help yourself move towards a more healthy lifestyle and tackle your mental health and obesity issues.

Now is the time to revisit all of those action plans and create one single plan for the next three months.

Using the template (**Appendix 2, page 138**) create a high-level plan showing what you want to achieve, how you are going to get there and the steps you will take along the way.

Then use the journal **(Appendix 3, page 139)** to record your progress every day for three months. Simply record your challenges, your triumphs and your thoughts along with any positive actions you have taken each day.

At the end of each week look back and see how well you have come and, if you have struggled, work out how you can do better next week.

The important thing is to keep moving forward towards your goals.

The Must Be More to Life Than This . . . ?

10: What is next for Steve?

Steve's Story Moving Forward

Ever since Ali and I started working on this book I have begun to feel excited about the future.

There is hope for people like me, struggling every day to get through yes but always looking forward to better times.

If this book changes a single negative attitude in just one person, then it will have been worth it. If this book helps just one person to re-evaluate their problems and make positive changes for the future, it will have been worth it.

I hope, with all my heart, that as you read through our book you come to understand a little more about the complex issues surrounding obesity.

I hope that you have used the interactive sections, the question and answer pages and thoughts capture sections to understand yourself better.

I hope that in drawing your own geo-emotional map of your relationship with food that you have made discoveries that will help you to overcome your issues in the future.

I am a work in progress. I know the road ahead is a difficult one and that it won't all come good overnight.

I will continue to lose weight and to help others through my podcast and the other voluntary work that I do. I will continue to spread the word, and I will never give up because I believe in me, and I believe in you too.

Every day I will be working on my podcast,

interviewing more people in the hope that by sharing our knowledge and experiences we can give hope to others who are struggling.

The world has been through a tough time recently. There cannot be many people who haven't been touched in some way by the Covid pandemic. You may have lost friends or loved ones; you may have been ill yourself.

Like Ali you may have been made redundant (although that turned out to be a great thing for her), and you may be struggling financially, with loneliness and even with the worry about what the future holds.

It's a scary world out there right now and there isn't much we can do about that, but I will say to you . . .

Be honest, be true, be kind and know that the journey will be worth it because . . .

There must be more to life than this . . .

Last Words for Inspiration

The new dawn blooms as we free it

For there is always light if only we are brave enough to see it

If only we are brave enough to be it

Amanda Gorman

You may say I'm a dreamer

But I'm not the only one

I hope someday you'll join us

And the world can live as one

John Lennon

But I know, somehow,

That it is only when it is dark enough

Can you see the stars

Martin Luther King Jr

Hope is that thing inside us that insists,

Despite all the evidence to the contrary,

That something better awaits us,

If we have the courage to reach for it,

And to fight for it and work for it

Barack Obama

Never give up, Have hope

Expect only the best from life

And take action to get it

Catherine Pulsifer

When you are at the end of your rope

Tie a knot and hold on

Theodore Roosevelt

Others may try to bring you down, pity them for they have their own issues

Your demons may rise to distract you from your path, ignore them for they have only their own interests at heart

Believe in yourself, every minute of every day, for you are the hero of your life story and only you can save yourself

Ali Bagley & Steve Beer

The Must Be More to Life Than This . . . ?

Appendices

1. Contact Details of Organisations & Support Groups

2. My Action Plan Template

3. My Three-Month Journal

4. Biography and Contact Details - Ali

5. Biography and Contact Details – Steve

6. A mention for our sponsors and supporters

7. References and Bibliography

Appendix 1: Contact Details of Organisations & Support Groups

HOOP UK	http://hoopuk.org.uk/
The National Centre for Eating Disorders	http://www.eating-disorders.org.uk/
NHS Obesity Information	https://www.nhs.uk/conditions/obesity/
NHS Social Care and Support Guide	https://www.nhs.uk/conditions/social-care-and-support-guide/
The National Centre for Eating Disorders	http://www.eating-disorders.org.uk/
The National Obesity Forum	http://www.nationalobesityforum.org.uk/
MaleVoiceED	http://www.malevoiced.com/
Overeaters Anonymous	http://www.oagb.org.uk/
Weight Concern	http://www.weightconcern.org.uk/
Weight Matters	https://www.weightmatters.co.uk/

Weight Wise	http://www.bdaweightwise.com/
The British Nutrition Foundation	http://www.nutrition.org.uk/

Appendix 2: Template for your Action Plan

Action	Benefit to Me	Step 1	Step 2	Step 3	Step 4	Date Achieved	Outcome
1							
2							
3							
4							
5							
6							
7							
8							
9							
10							

My Action Plan Template

Appendix 3: My Three-Month Journal

Use the following pages to record and track your progress every day.

Keep in mind that every day is a new day, no matter what happened the day before.

Review your journal each week and congratulate yourself for every success.

Never punish yourself when things go wrong. Simply learn from them and move on.

Re-visit your Geo-Emotional map any time that you need to. It is a living document and you can re-draw and update it whenever you want to.

MY DAILY JOURNAL

. . . on my road to a healthier lifestyle

Week 1: week commencing _____

Monday

_____
_____
_____

Tuesday

_____
_____
_____

Wednesday

_____
_____
_____

Thursday

_____
_____
_____

Friday

_____
_____
_____

Saturday & Sunday

_____
_____
_____
_____
_____

MY DAILY JOURNAL
. . . on my road to a healthier lifestyle

Week 2: week commencing _____

Monday

_____

_____

_____

Tuesday

_____

_____

_____

Wednesday

_____

_____

_____

Thursday

_____

_____

_____

Friday

_____

_____

_____

Saturday & Sunday

_____

_____

_____

_____

_____

MY DAILY JOURNAL

. . . on my road to a healthier lifestyle

Week 3: week commencing _____

Monday

_____

_____

_____

Tuesday

_____

_____

_____

Wednesday

_____

_____

_____

Thursday

_____

_____

_____

Friday

_____

_____

_____

Saturday & Sunday

_____

_____

_____

_____

_____

MY DAILY JOURNAL

. . . on my road to a healthier lifestyle

Week 4: week commencing _____

Monday

_____

_____

_____

Tuesday

_____

_____

_____

Wednesday

_____

_____

_____

Thursday

_____

_____

_____

Friday

_____

_____

_____

Saturday & Sunday

_____

_____

_____

_____

_____

MY DAILY JOURNAL

. . . on my road to a healthier lifestyle

Week 5: week commencing _____

Monday

_____

_____

_____

Tuesday

_____

_____

_____

Wednesday

_____

_____

_____

Thursday

_____

_____

_____

Friday

_____

_____

_____

Saturday & Sunday

_____

_____

_____

_____

_____

MY DAILY JOURNAL

. . . on my road to a healthier lifestyle

Week 6: week commencing _____

Monday

_____

_____

_____

Tuesday

_____

_____

_____

Wednesday

_____

_____

_____

Thursday

_____

_____

_____

Friday

_____

_____

_____

Saturday & Sunday

_____

_____

_____

_____

_____

MY DAILY JOURNAL

. . . on my road to a healthier lifestyle

Week 7: week commencing _____

Monday

_____
_____
_____

Tuesday

_____
_____
_____

Wednesday

_____
_____
_____

Thursday

_____
_____
_____

Friday

_____
_____
_____

Saturday & Sunday

_____
_____
_____
_____
_____

MY DAILY JOURNAL

. . . on my road to a healthier lifestyle

Week 8: week commencing _____

Monday

_____

_____

_____

Tuesday

_____

_____

_____

Wednesday

_____

_____

_____

Thursday

_____

_____

_____

Friday

_____

_____

_____

Saturday & Sunday

_____

_____

_____

_____

MY DAILY JOURNAL

. . . on my road to a healthier lifestyle

Week 9: week commencing _____

Monday

_____

_____

_____

Tuesday

_____

_____

_____

Wednesday

_____

_____

_____

Thursday

_____

_____

_____

Friday

_____

_____

_____

Saturday & Sunday

_____

_____

_____

_____

_____

MY DAILY JOURNAL

. . . on my road to a healthier lifestyle

Week 10: week commencing _____

Monday

_____
_____
_____

Tuesday

_____
_____
_____

Wednesday

_____
_____
_____

Thursday

_____
_____
_____

Friday

_____
_____
_____

Saturday & Sunday

_____
_____
_____
_____
_____

MY DAILY JOURNAL

. . . on my road to a healthier lifestyle

Week 11: week commencing _____

Monday

_____

_____

_____

Tuesday

_____

_____

_____

Wednesday

_____

_____

_____

Thursday

_____

_____

_____

Friday

_____

_____

_____

Saturday & Sunday

_____

_____

_____

_____

_____

MY DAILY JOURNAL

. . . on my road to a healthier lifestyle

Week 12: week commencing _____

Monday

_____

_____

_____

Tuesday

_____

_____

_____

Wednesday

_____

_____

_____

Thursday

_____

_____

_____

Friday

_____

_____

_____

Saturday & Sunday

_____

_____

_____

_____

_____

MY DAILY JOURNAL

. . . on my road to a healthier lifestyle

Week 13: week commencing _____

Monday

_____

_____

_____

Tuesday

_____

_____

_____

Wednesday

_____

_____

_____

Thursday

_____

_____

_____

Friday

_____

_____

_____

Saturday & Sunday

_____

_____

_____

_____

_____

MY DAILY JOURNAL

. . . on my road to a healthier lifestyle

MY GOALS FOR THE NEXT THREE MONTHS

Weight Loss

_____

_____

_____

Exercise

_____

_____

_____

Mindfulness

_____

_____

_____

Good Habits

_____

_____

_____

Relationships

_____

_____

_____

Other

_____

_____

_____

_____

Appendix 4: Biography and Contact Details - Ali

Ali Bagley is a Business Impact and Writers Coach, An Amazon number 1 bestselling Author, Director of an International Coaching Platform and a Geographer of Emotions.

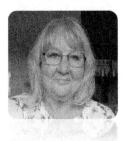

Her background is in project and proposals management however, aged 56, at the start of the Covid pandemic, Ali decided that life was too short to waste in a toxic corporate environment, so she took redundancy, re-trained as a certified coach and has not looked back since.

"All my life, the times I have been happiest and most fulfilled have been when my work has involved helping people". Ali was a Weight Watchers Coach for 6 years in her thirties and it was the life changing results she saw in her clients then, that convinced her to get back into a coaching role.

In October 2020 Ali met Marco Bertagni, the visionary developer of the geo-emotional mapping methodology that she now uses in all of her coaching. "That meeting changed the course of my life and my business. We now work together bringing emotional geography to the world through multiple courses, journeys and games."

Since starting her business Ali has written and published several 'how to' and business support books, both individually, in collaboration with others, and as editor and publisher for others. All the books are available on Amazon and include:

The Coaches Resource Directory – Ali Bagley -
Oct 2020
https://www.amazon.co.uk/dp/B08L4GML6J

Nailing Your Niche – Ali Bagley -
Oct 2020
https://www.amazon.co.uk/dp/B08LNPTD7X

Planning to Inspire, The Coaches Essential
Handbook and Planner – Ali Bagley & Victoria
Morley - Feb 2021
https://www.amazon.co.uk/dp/B08WYC8QZL

Inspirational Planning, The Business Owners
Handbook and Planner – Ali Bagley & Victoria
Morley - Feb 2021
https://www.amazon.co.uk/dp/B08WZHBKD1

Find Your Place Hygge Journal – Victoria Morley
– Mar 2021
https://www.amazon.co.uk/dp/B08YQCQ87W

My Accountability Journal, day by day progress
towards my goals – Ali Bagley & Ian George – Mar
2021
https://www.amazon.co.uk/dp/B08YS622XH

The River of Life – Marco Bertagni – May 2021
https://www.amazon.co.uk/dp/B09444VP1G

Love Coaching, Hate Business (Amazon No1
Bestseller) – Ali Bagley & Susan Lane – Sept 2021
https://www.amazon.co.uk/dp/B09CQG6V5G

Burnout to Bold, Fom a Flickering Light to a Bold
Flame – Marie Jenkins – Oct 2021
https://www.amazon.co.uk/dp/B09F1KNM84

What Will Charlie & Teddy Do Today (a childrens
book) – Alison Bagley – Dec 2020
https://www.amazon.co.uk/dp/B08P5Q6TT1

Ali also runs a number of courses that support writers, business owners and individuals looking to grow and develop both in business and life. Here are a few:

Think Mood, Not Food, shifting your mindset for mental and physical wellbeing in a creative and inspirational way, for busy women over 40:
https://alibagleycoach.samcart.com/products/mood-not-food

Everything You Need to Know About Online Course Development, for coaches and business owners who want to share knowledge and grow their business:
https://alibagleycoach.samcart.com/products/everyt hing-you-need-to-know-about-online-course-development-recorded

How to Build a Practical and Resilient Business Foundation, a comprehensive course for new business owners:
https://alibagleycoach.samcart.com/products/how-to-build-a-practical-and-resilient-business-foundation-

How to Get the Writing Skills You Need to Grow Your Business, from posts, to blogs to book creation:
https://alibagleycoach.samcart.com/products/how-to-develop-your-writing-skills-to-grow-your-business

Re-Vamp, how to make your home your castle on a budget:
https://alibagleycoach.samcart.com/products/re-vamp

Last but not least, Ali works one to one on a bespoke basis with individuals and businesses to develop their writing projects, develop their business plans and strategies and develop collaboration in teams.

Through her business, **Ali Bagley Coaching**, Ali has worked with clients all over the world to develop their online courses, write and publish their books and grow their businesses.

If you would like to know more about Ali's books, courses and one to one services, or learn more about emotional geography as a tool for your own self-development or for your business please contact her directly by emailing her at:

ali@alibagleycoaching.co.uk

or

ali@emotional-geography.com

You can also visit her website:

https://www.comgortcornerwithali.com

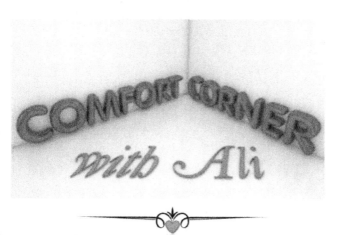

Appendix 5: Biography and Contact Details - Steve

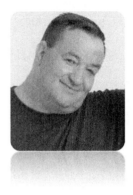

Steve Beer is the creator and host of Crossroads Podcast UK.

He has struggled with obesity for 20 years, suffering verbal and physical abuse in the street and vilification on TV and in the newspapers.

Happily married now to his 6th wife Michelle, he has turned his life around by helping others through his podcast, his work as an ambassador for obesity awareness and through his church and local council voluntary work.

Steve still has an uphill battle to win with his weight, a battle he is determined to win, yet as he fights on his first thought is still to help others in a similar place.

A devout Christian he believes that it is his faith that has kept him going, even when he was on the brink of taking his own life.

If you would like to be a guest on Steve's podcast or would like more information about his voluntary work you can contact him at: stephenbeer40@yahoo.com or visit the podcast FaceBook page at: https://www.facebook.com/groups/7555076553705 73

Appendix 6: A mention for our supporters

Thank you to Marco Bertagni, founder and visionary of Emotional-Geography UK Limited. It is Marco's methodology for Geo-Emotional Mapping that has helped Ali and so many others to re-evaluate, understand and develop solutions to problems that have been both permanent and positively life changing.

Thank you to everyone who has been a guest or tuned in to the Crossroads UK Podcast. We hope that you continue to listen, enjoy and share our broadcasts.

When Ali Bagley said she would help me to write this book it was an answer to my prayer. Thank you Lord, and thank you Ali for your patience and hard work in getting this done. You will never know how happy you have made me.

Thank you to Brixington Church for accepting me and Michelle with special thanks to Maria, Andrew, Sue and Michelle M for your help.

And last but most importantly, thank you to my darling wife Michelle who has been with me and there for me through it all, and my Dad Bob, I love you both loads xxx

Appendix 7: References and Bibliography

Statistics on obesity in the UK were sourced from:https://files.digital.nhs.uk/9D/4195D5/HSE19-Overweight-obesity-rep.pdf

and

https://digital.nhs.uk/data-and-information/publications/statistical/statistics-on-obesity-physical-activity-and-diet

and

Hospital Episode Statistics (HES), NHS Digital and include data published on 18th May 2021 covering a period from 1st April 2019 to 31st December 2020.

'Why Diets Don't Work', Maureen Moerbeck of Nutritionist Resource: https://www.nutritionist-resource.org.uk/blog/2020/10/02/why-diets-dont-work

The Health Survey for England 2019: https://files.digital.nhs.uk/9D/4195D5/HSE19-Overweight-obesity-rep.pdf

The Daily Mile initiative. https://thedailymile.co.uk/

Measures to prevent childhood obesity: www.eufic.org

The Priory Group UK: https://www.priorygroup.com/blog/the-relationship-between-mental-health-and-obesity

Public Health England reports and statistics:
https://www.gov.uk/government/organisations/publi
c-health-england

Tackling obesity: empowering adults and children
to live healthier lives'
https://www.gov.uk/government/publications/tacklin
g-obesity-government-strategy/tackling-obesity-
empowering-adults-and-children-to-live-healthier-
lives

Information on the government initiative towards
sugar reduction sourced from:
https://www.gov.uk/government/collections/sugar-
reduction

Childhood obesity: a plan for action
https://www.gov.uk/government/publications/childh
ood-obesity-a-plan-for-action

Obesity Action – Is there a link between mental
health and obesity:
https://www.obesityaction.org/community/article-
library/obesity-and-mental-health-is-there-a-link/

www.healthexpress.co.uk/obesity/uk-statistics

Relationships statistics sourced from:
https://review42.com/uk

Mind, the mental health charity – Obesity and
Mental Health: https://mindcharity.co.uk/wp-
content/uploads/2016/03/Obesity-and-Mental-
Health.pdf

Merrill Littleberry, Obesity and Mental Health, is there a link?:
https://www.obesityaction.org/community/article-library/obesity-and-mental-health-is-there-a-link/

NHS Statistics, drug use in young people:
https://digital.nhs.uk/data-and-information/publications/statistical/statistics-on-drug-misuse/2019/part-4-drug-use-among-young-people

Government report on young peoples substance abuse:
https://www.gov.uk/government/statistics/substance-misuse-treatment-for-young-people-statistics-2019-to-2020/young-peoples-substance-misuse-treatment-statistics-2019-to-2020-report

Young Minds, the mental health charity:
https://www.youngminds.org.uk/young-person/coping-with-life/drugs-and-alcohol/

'The Social Dilemma: Social Media and Your Mental Health': https://www.mcleanhospital.org/

'Is there a link between obesity and mental health': https://www.iser.essex.ac.uk/

Obesity statistics:
www.healthexpress.co.uk/obesity/uk-statistics

Association of Adiposity and Mental Health Functioning across the Lifespan: Findings from Understanding Society (The UK Household Longitudinal Study):
http://journals.plos.org/plosone/article?id=10.1371/journal.pone.0148561

Think Mood Not Food: the lifestyle change program:
https://alibagleycoach.samcart.com/products/mood-not-food

CIPD (The professional body for HR and people development - https://www.cipd.co.uk/

5 Ways Hope Impacts Health and Happiness (5 ways the science of hope influences the way you work and life), Paula Davis J.D. M.A.P.P 2013, https://www.psychologytoday.com/us/blog/pressure-proof/201303/5-ways-hope-impacts-health-happiness

the podcast host:
(https://www.thepodcasthost.com/)

The Must Be More to Life Than This . . . ?

THERE MUST BE MORE TO LIFE THAN THIS . . . ?

One man's journey on the human side of the statistics and attitudes surrounding obesity in the UK today

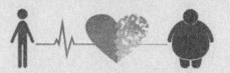

STEVE BEER & ALI BAGLEY

Printed in Great Britain
by Amazon